W0227936

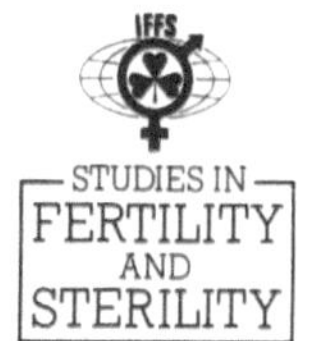

In Vitro Fertilization, Embryo Transfer and Early Pregnancy

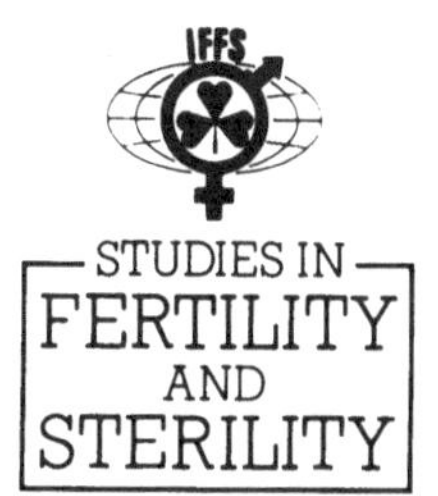

STUDIES IN
FERTILITY
AND
STERILITY

In Vitro Fertilization, Embryo Transfer and Early Pregnancy

Edited by
R.F. Harrison, J. Bonnar
and W. Thompson

Themes from the XIth World Congress on Fertility and Sterility, Dublin, June 1983, held under the Auspices of the International Federation of Fertility Societies

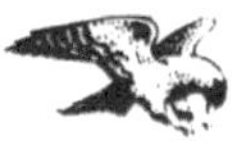 SPRINGER SCIENCE+BUSINESS MEDIA, LLC 

Published in the UK and Europe by
MTP Press Limited
Falcon House
Lancaster, England

British Library Cataloguing in Publication Data

World Congress on Fertility and Sterility
(11th : 1983 : Dublin)
In vitro fertilization, embryo transfer and early pregnancy.—
(Studies in fertility and sterility)
1. Fertilization in vitro
I. Title II. Harrison, R.F. III. Bonnar, J.
IV. Thompson, William, *1937–*
V. International Federation of Fertility Societies
VI. Series 599.033'33 RG135

ISBN 978-94-011-8134-1 ISBN 978-94-011-8132-7 (eBook)
DOI 10.1007/978-94-011-8132-7

Library of Congress Cataloging in Publication Data

Main entry under title:
In vitro fertilization, embryo transfer, and early pregnancy.
(Studies in fertility and sterility)
Bibliography: p.
Includes index.
1. Fertilization in vitro – Congresses. 2.Embryo transplantation – Congresses. 3. pregnancy – Congresses. I. Harrison, R.F. (Robert Frederick) II. Bonnar, John. III. Thompson, W. IV.World Congress of Fertility and Sterility (11th : 1983 : Dublin, Dublin) V. International Federation of Fertility Societies. VI. Series.
[DNLM: 1. Fertilization In Vitro – congresses. 2. Embryo Transfer – congresses. 3. Pregnancy – congresses. W3 W0542 12th 1983i / WQ 205 W927 1983i]
QP2733.15 1984 618.1'78 84–11242
ISBN 978-94-011-8134-1

Phototypesetting by
David John Services Ltd, Maidenhead

Contents

PART III: SEMEN AND SPERMATOZOA

Section 1: Animal Studies

Section 2: Practical Aspects of Human Semen Quality

PART IV: *IN VITRO* FERTILIZATION AND EMBRYO TRANSFER. CLINICAL RESULTS

Section 1: In Humans

Preface

In Vitro Fertilization, Embryo Transfer and Early Pregnancy is undoubtably the most exciting and onwardly progressing field in reproductive medicine today. It forms the major subject matter of this the second volume of the Proceedings and the first book of Related Communication papers given at the XI International Federation of Fertility Societies World Congress on Fertility and Sterility held in Dublin, Ireland from June 26th to July 1st 1983.

The papers have been grouped into closely allied topics covering sequentially in three parts: Follicle and Ovum in the Human, Follicle and Ovum in the Animal Model, and Semen and Spermatozoa. Preceding a timely reminder on Ethical and Legal Aspects of IVF are some of the remarkable clinical results now been obtained throughout the world. The final section concerns various aspects of Pregnancy in Animals and Humans and is included in this volume because of its close relationship to the main subject matter.

Related Communications sessions often produce the largest amounts of up-to-date information to be given on a particular subject during a Congress. IFFS Dublin '83 proved to be no exception. So although scientific and medical endeavour will ensure that knowledge and progress in the field will soom overtake many of the conclusions reached in these papers, nevertheless we hope you will agree in the merit of producing such a record of the state of the art at this time.

Robert F. Harrison
John Bonnar
William Thompson

Dublin 1983.

List of Contributors

G. ACKER
Unité n 187, INSERM
32 Rue des Carnets
94.140 Clamart
FRANCE

S. AL HASANI
Klinik für Frauenheilkunde und Geburtshilfe I und II
der Medizinishen Hoschschule Lübeck
Ratzeburger Allee 160
D-2400 Lübeck
WEST GERMANY

S. AVERY
Dr. B.A. Mason's Clinic
London W1N 3FJ
UNITED KINGDOM

C. AZUMA
Department of Obstetrics and Gynecology
Osaka University Medical School
1-1-50 Fukushima
Fukushimaku
Osaka 553
JAPAN

M. BARTHEL
Universitäts-Frauenklinik Erlangen
Universitätsstrasse 21-23
D-8520 Erlangen
WEST GERMANY

V. BAUKLOH
Institute for Hormone and Fertility Disorders
Lornsenstrasse 4
D-2000 Hamburg 50
WEST GERMANY

P.D. BROMWICH
Department of Obstetrics and Gynaecology
University of Birmingham
Birmingham Maternity Hospital
Queen Elizabeth Medical Centre
Birmingham B15 2TG
UNITED KINGDOM

D. ČECHOVÁ
Department of Biochemistry
Institute of Molecular Genetics
Czechoslovak Academy of Sciences
Flemingovo nám. 2
166 10 Prague 6
CZECHOSLOVAKIA

C.M. CHIA
Department of Obstetrics and Gynaecology
National University of Singapore
Kandang Kerbau Hospital
Hampshire Road
SINGAPORE 0821

M.R.N. DARLING
Rotunda Hospital
Dublin 1
IRELAND

G.G. DE SCHEPPER
Institute of Human Genetics
University of Amsterdam
Sarphatistraat 217
1018 BX Amsterdam
THE NETHERLANDS

G.U. DETLEFSEN
Department of Gynecology
Bispebjerg Hospital
Bispebjerg Bakke
DK-2400 Copenhagen NV
DENMARK

K. DIEDERICH
Klinik für Frauenheilkunde und Geburtshilfe I und II der Medizinischen
Hochschule Lübeck
Ratzeburger Allee 160
D-2400 Lübeck
WEST GERMANY

R.G. EDWARDS
Bourn Hall, Bourn
Cambridge
UNITED KINGDOM

S.A.F. EL-MOUGY
Department of Physiology
Faculty of Veterinary Medicine
Zagazig University
Zagazig
EGYPT

Y. ENDO
Department of Obstetrics and Gynecology
School of Medicine,
Keio University
35 Shinaromachi, Shinjuku-ku
Tokyo 160
JAPAN

T. ENDOH
Department of Obstetrics and Gynecology
Sapporo Medical College
South 1, West 16
Chuo-ku, Sapporo
Hokkaido
JAPAN

F. FISCHL
2nd Department of Gynecology and Obstetrics
University of Vienna
Spitalgasse 23
A-1090 Vienna
AUSTRIA

Y. FUMITA
Department of Obstetrics and Gynecology
Osaka University Medical School
1-1-50 Fukushima
Fukushimaku, Osaka 553
JAPAN

P. FYLLING
Department of Gynaecology
Ullevaal Hospital
Oslo 2
NORWAY

J.G. GRUDZINSKAS
Department of Obstetrics and Gynaecology
The London Hospital
Whitechapel
London
UNITED KINGDOM

U. HAMERICH
Klinik für Frauenheilkunde und Geburtshilfe I und II
der Medizinischen Hochscule Lübeck
Ratzebruger Allee 160
D-2400 Lübeck
WEST GERMANY

A. HANADA
3rd Department of Reproduction
National Institute of Animal Industry
PO Box 5, 2 Ikenodai
Kukizaki, Inashiki
Ibaraki 305
JAPAN

A. HASEGAWA
Department of Obstetrics and Gynecology
Hyogo Medical College
1-1 Mukogawa-cho
Nishinomiya 663
JAPAN

M. HASHIMOTO
Department of Obstetrics and Gynecology
Sapporo Medical College
South 1, West 16
Chuo-ku, Sapporo
Hokkaido
JAPAN

K. HATA
Mitsubishi Yuka Medical Science
1-2-10 Narimasu
Itabashi-ku
Tokyo 175
JAPAN

J.T. HAZEKAMP
Department of Gynaecology
Ullevaal Hospital
Oslo 2
NORWAY

P. HERNUSS
Fertility-Center, Vienna
Formanekgasse 57
A-1190 Vienna
AUSTRIA

H.A. HESHMAT
Department of Physiology
Faculty of Veterinary Medicine
Zagazig University
Zagazig
EGYPT

Y. HIRAI
Department of Biochemistry II
Nippon Medical School
1-1-5 Sendagi, Bunkyo-ku
Tokyo
JAPAN 113

M. HIRANO
Department of Obstetrics and Gynecology
Tohoku University School of Medicine
Seiryo-machi, Sendai 980
JAPAN

A. HØISETH
Department of Radiology
Ullevaal Hospital
Oslo 2
NORWAY

H.O. HOPPEN
Max-Planck-Institut für Experimentelle Endokrinologie
D-3000 Hannover
WEST GERMANY

H. HOSHIAI
Department of Obstetrics and Gynecology
Tohoku University School of Medicine
Seiryo-machi, Sendai 980
JAPAN

J. HUBER
1st University Clinic of Obstetrics and Gynecology
Spitalgasse 23
A-1090 Vienna
AUSTRIA

P. HUSSLEIN
1st University Clinic of Obstetrics and Gynecology
Spitalgasse 23
A-1090 Vienna
AUSTRIA

R. IIZUKA
Department of Obstetrics and Gynecology
School of Medicine
Keio University
35 Shinanomachi, Shinjuku-ku
Tokyo 160
JAPAN

O. ISHIHARA
Department of Obstetrics and Gynecology
Faculty of Medicine
University of Tokyo
7-3-1 Hongo, Bunkyo-ku
Tokyo 113
JAPAN

S. ISOJIMA
Department of Obstetrics and Gynecology
Hyogo Medical College
1-1 Mukogawa-cho
Nishinomiya
663 JAPAN

A. IWAKI
2nd Department of Gynecology and Obstetrics
School of Medicine
Toho University
Ohashi Hospital
2-17-6 Ohadhi, Meguro-ku
Tokyo
JAPAN

H. JANISCH
2nd Department of Gynecology and Obstetrics
University of Vienna
Spitalgasse 23
A-1090 Vienna
AUSTRIA

V. JONÁKOVÁ
Department of Biochemistry
Institute of Molecular Genetics
Czechoslovak Academy of Sciences
Flemingovo nám. 2
166 10 Prague 6
CZECHOSLOVAKIA

M. JONDET
Fondation de Recherche en Hormonologie
26 Boulevard Brune
75014 Paris
FRANCE

Y. KANEKO
Kanda 2nd Clinic
3-20-14 Nishi-Azabu
Minato-ku
Tokyo 106
JAPAN

H. KANZAKI
Department of Gynecology and Obstetrics
Faculty of Medicine
Kyoto University
54 Shogoin Kawahara-cho
Sakyo-ku
Kyoto 606
JAPAN

H. KARLIC
1st University Clinic of Obstetrics and Gynecology
Spitalgasse 23
A-1090 Vienna
AUSTRIA

H. KASEKI
Department of Biochemistry II
Nippon Medical School
1-1-5 Sendagi, Bunkyo-ku
Tokyo
JAPAN 113

T. KASEKI
Department of Fertility and Sterility
Kaseki Maternity Hospital
4-16-16 Sakae, Naka-ku
Nagoya
JAPAN 460

M. KATO
2nd Department of Anatomy
School of Medicine
Toho University
Ohashi Hospital
2-17-6 Ohadhi, Meguro-ku
Tokyo
JAPAN

N. KAWAMURA
Department of Gynecology and Obstetrics
Faculty of Medicine
Kyoto University
54 Shogoin Kawahara-cho
Sakyo-ku, Kyoto 606
JAPAN

F. KAYAMA
Department of Obstetrics and Gynecology
University of Tokyo
7-3-1 Hongo, Bunkyo-ku
Tokyo 113
JAPAN

H. KEY
Dr. B.A. Mason's Clinic
25 Weymouth Street
London W1N 3FJ
UNITED KINGDOM

K. KINOSHITA
Department of Obstetrics and Gynecology
Faculty of Medicine
University of Tokyo
7-3-1 Hongo, Bunkyo-ku
Tokyo 113
JAPAN

T. KINOSHITA
2nd Department of Gynecology and Obstetrics
School of Medicine
Toho University
Ohashi Hospital
2-17-6 Ohadhi, Megwo-ku
Tokyo
JAPAN

W. KNOGLER
1st University Clinic of Obstetrics and Gynecology
Spitalgasse 23
A-1090 Vienna
AUSTRIA

E. KOJIMA
Kanda 2nd Clinic
3-20-14 Nishi-Azabu
Minato-ku
Tokyo 106
JAPAN

I. KOSKIMIES
II Department of Obstetrics and Gynecology
Helsinki University Central Hospital
Haarmanink 3
00290 Helsinki 29
FINLAND

K. KOYAMA
Department of Obstetrics and Gynecology
Hyogo Medical College
1-1 Mukogawa-cho
Nishinomiya 663
JAPAN

F. KRASSNIGG
Andrology Unit
Department oif Dermatology
University of Munich
Frauenlobstrasse 9-11
D-8000 München 2
WEST GERMANY

D. KREBS
Klinik für Frauenheilkunde und Geburtshilfe
I und II der Medizinischen Hochschule Lübeck
Ratzeburger Allee 160
D-2400 Lübeck
WEST GERMANY

E. KUBISTA
1st University Clinic of Obstetrics and Gynecology
Spitalgasse 23
A-1090 Vienna
AUSTRIA

K. KURACHI
Department of Obstetrics and Gynecology
Osaka University Medical School
1-1-50 Fukushima, Fukushimaki
Osaka 553
JAPAN

S. KURASAWA
Department of Obstetrics and Gynecology
School of Medicine
Keio University
35 Shinanomachi, Shinjuku-ku
Tokyo 160
JAPAN

H.Y. LAW
Department of Obstetrics and Gynaecology
National University of Singapore
Kandang Kerbau Hospital
Hampshire Road
SINGAPORE 0821

P.E. LEBECH
Department of Obstetrics and Gynecology
Frederiksberg Hospital
DK-2000 Copenhagen F
DENMARK

F. LEHMANN
Klinik für Frauenheilkunde und Geburtshilfe I und II
der Medizinischen Hochschule Lübeck
Ratzeburger Allee 160
02400 Lübeck
WEST GERMANY

D.J. LITTLE
Department of Obstetrics and Gynaecology
University of Birmingham
Birmingham Maternity Hospital
Queen Elizabeth Medical Centre
Birmingham B15 2TG
UNITED KINGDOM

S. LIUKKONEN
I Department of Obstetrics and Gynecology
Helsinki University Central Hospital
Haartmanink 3
00290 Helsinki 29
FINLAND

V. MAASSEN
Department of Obstetrics and Gynaecology
Free University of Berlin
Charlottenburg
WEST GERMANY

S. MACKABE
Kanda 2nd Clinic
3-20-14 Nishi-Azabu
Minato-ku
Tokyo 106
JAPAN

A.M. MACKEN
Department of Obstetrics and Gynaecology
University of Birmingham
Birmingham Maternity Hospital
Queen Elizabeth Medical Centre
Birmingham N15 2TG
UNITED KINGDOM

L. METTLER
Universitäts-Frauenklinik
Michaels Hebammenlehranstalt
Hegeurschstrasse 4
D-2300 Kiel 1
WEST GERMANY

Y. MINAGAWA
Department of Obstetrics and Gynecology
Osaka University Medical School
1-1-50 Fukushima, Fukushimaku
Osaka 553
JAPAN

K. MIYAZAKI
Department of Obstetrics and Gynecology
Osaka Medical College
2-7 Daigakucho, Takatsuki
Osaka 569
JAPAN

M. MIZUNO
Department of Obstetrics and Gynecology
University of Tokyo
7-3-1 Hongo, Bunkyo-ku
Tokyo 113
JAPAN

K. MOMOSE
Kanda 2nd Clinic
3-20-14 Nishi-Azabu
Minato-ku
Tokyo 106
JAPAN

R. MORI
Department of Obstetrics and Gynecology
Tohoku University
School of Medicine
Seiryo-machi, Sendai 980
JAPAN

Y. MORITA
Department of Obstetrics and Gynecology
University of Tokyo
7-3-1 Hongo, Bunkyo-ku
Tokyo 113
JAPAN

J. MÜLLER
Universitäts-Frauenklinik Erlangen
Universitätsstrasse 21-23
8520 Erlangen
WEST GERMANY

E. MÜLLER-TYL
2nd Department of Gynecology and Obstetrics
University of Vienna
A-1090 Vienna
AUSTRIA

L. MYATT
Institute of Obstetrics and Gynaecology
Hammersmith Hospital
London W12 0HS
UNITED KINGDOM

T. NAGAE
2nd Department of Gynecology and Obstetrics
School of Medicine
Toho University
Ohashi Hospital
2-17-6 Ohadhi, Meguro-ku
Tokyo
JAPAN

F. NAGAIKE
Department of Obstetrics and Gynecology
Tohoku University
School of Medicing
Seiryo-machi, Sendai 980
JAPAN

K. NAKAMURO
Department of Obstetrics and Gynecology
Osake University Medical School
1-1-50 Fukushima, Fukushimaku
Osaka 553
JAPAN

T. NEMOTO
Nemoto Maternity Clinic
2-26-16 Gyotoku-ekimae
Ichikawa-shi, Chiba Pref.
JAPAN 270-01

J.R. NEWTON
Department of Obstetrics and Gynaecology
University of Birmingham
Birmingham Maternity Hospital
Queen Elizabeth Medical Centre
Birmingham B15 2TG
UNITED KINGDOM

S.C. NG
Department of Obstetrics and Gynaecology
National University of Singapore
Kandang Kerbau Hospital
Hampshire Road
SINGAPORE 0821

K. NOKUBI
2nd Department of Anatomy
School of Medicine
Toho University
Ohashi Hospital
2-17-6 Ohadhi, Meguro-ku
Tokyo
JAPAN

A. OKADA
2nd Department of Anatomy
School of Medicine
Toho University
Ohashi Hospital
2-17-6 Ohadhi, Meguro-ku
Tokyo
JAPAN

H. OKAMURA
Department of Gynecology and Obstetrics
Faculty of Medicine
Kyoto University
54 Shogoin Kawahara-cho
Sakyo-ku, Kyoto 606
JAPAN

Y. OKUDA
Department of Gynecology and Obstetrics
Faculty of Medicine
Kyoto University
54 Shogoin Kawahara-cho
Sakyo-ku, Kyoto 606
JAPAN

G. OMURA
Kanda 2nd Clinic
3-20-14 Nishi-Azabu
Minato-ku
Tokyo 106
JAPAN

B. OTTESEN
Department of Obstetrics and Gynecology
Frederiksberg Hospital
57 N.Fasanvej
DK-2000 Copenhagen F
DENMARK

S. PAUL
Human Reproduction Unit
Department of Obstetrics and Gynecology
University of Kiel
Hegewischstrasse 4
D-2300 Kiel
WEST GERMANY

S.C. PEDERSEN
Department of Gynecology
Bispebjerg Hospital
Bispebjerg Bakke
DK-2400 Copenhagen NV
DENMARK

Y.M. RADWAN
Department of Physiology
Faculty of Veterinary Medicine
Zagazig University
Zagazig
EGYPT

S.S. RATNAM
Department of Obstetrics and Gynaecology
National University of Singapore
Kandang Kerbau Hospital
Hampshire Road
SINGAPORE 0821

M. RAUFF
Department of Obstetrics and Gynaecology
National University of Singapore
Kandang Kerbau Hospital
Hampshire Road
SINGAPORE 0821

H.-H. RIEDEL
Human Reproduction Unit
Department of Obstetrics and Gynecology
University of Kiel
Hegewischstrasse 4
D-2300 Kiel
WEST GERMANY

F. SAJI
Department of Obstetrics and Gynecology
Osaka University Medical School
1-1-50 Fukushima, Fukushimaku
Osaka 553
JAPAN

S. SAKAMOTO
Department of Obstetrics and Gynecology
Faculty of Medicine
University of Tokyo
7-3-1 Hongo, Bunkyo-ku
Tokyo 113
JAPAN

P. SARTOR
Neurophysiologie Groupe Metricité
Université de Bordeaux II
146 Rue Les Saignet
33076 Bordeaux Cédex
FRANCE

KODO SATO
Department of Obstetrics and Gynecology
University of Tokyo
7-3-1 Hongo, Bunkyo-ku
Tokyo 113
JAPAN

KUMIKO SATO
Department of Biochemistry II
Nippon Medical School
1-1-5 Sendagi, Bunkyo-ku
Tokyo
JAPAN 113

K. SATOH
Department of Obstetrics and Gynecology
Faculty of Medicine
University of Tokyo
7-3-1 Hongo, Bunkyo-ku
Tokyo 113
JAPAN

T. SATOH
Department of Obstetrics and Gynecology
Sapporo Medical College
South 1, West 16
Chuo-ku, Sapporo
Hokkaido
JAPAN

M. SAUNDERS
Department of Obstetrics and Gynaecology
Royal North Shore Hospital of Sydney
St Leonards
New South Wales 2065
AUSTRALIA

J.G. SCHENKER
Department of Obstetrics and Gynecology
Hadassah University Hospital
Jerusalem 91 120
ISRAEL

L. SCHIERUP
Department of Gynecology and Obstetrics
Nykøbing Fl. Centralsygehus
15 Fjordvej
DK-4800 Nykøbing Falster
DENMARK

W.B. SCHILL
Andrology Unit
Department of Dermatology
University of Munich
Frauenlobstrasse 9-11
D-8000 München 2
WEST GERMANY

W. SCHNEIDER
1st University Clinic of Obstetrics and Gynecology
Spitalgasse 23
A-1090 Vienna
AUSTRIA

R. SCHOLLER
Fondation de Recherche en Hormonologie
26 Boulevard Brune
75014 Paris
FRANCE

CHR. SCHULZ
Klinik für Frauenheilkunde und Geburtshilfe I und II der Medizinischen Hochschule Lübeck
Ratzeburger Allee 160
D-2400 Lübeck
WEST GERMANY

K. SEMM
Department of Obstetrics and Gynecology
University of Kiel
Hegewischstrasse 4
23 Kiel 1
WEST GERMANY

M.J. SINOSICH
Department of Obstetrics and Gynecology
University of Kiel
Hegewischstrasse 4
23 Kiel 1
WEST GERMANY

M.J. SINOSICH
Department of Obstetrics and Gynaecology
Royal North Shore Hospital of Sydney
St. Leonards
New South Wales 2065
AUSTRALIA

F. SØNDERGAARD
Department of Gynecology and Obstetrics
Frederiksberg Hospital
57 N. Fasanvej
DK-2000 Copenhagen F
DENMARK

H. SPIELMANN
Department of Obstetrics and Gynaecology
Free University of Berlin
Charlottenburg
WEST GERMANY

C. STADLER
Department of Obstetrics and Gynaecology
Free University of Berlin
Charlottenburg
WEST GERMANY

M. STAUBER
Department of Obstretrics and Gynaecology
Free University of Berlin
Charlottenburg
WEST GERMANY

R.P. STAVES
Universitäts-Frauenklinik
Michaelis Hebammenlehranstalt
Hegewischstrasses 4
D-2300 Kiel 1
WEST GERMANY

K. SUGAWARA
Department of Chemistry
Nippon Medical School
2-297-2 Kosugi-cho
Nakahara-ku
Kawaski
JAPAN 211

O. SUGIMOTO
Department of Obstetrics and Gynecology
Osaka Medical College
2-7 Daigakucho, Takatsuki
Osaka
569 JAPAN

M. SUZUKI
Department of Obstetrics and Gynecology
Tohoku University School of Medicine
Seiryo-machi
Sendai 980
JAPAN

S. SUZUKI
Department of Obstetrics and Gynecology
School of Medicine
Keio University
35 Shinanomachi, Shinjuku-ku
Tokyo 169
JAPAN

S. SZALAY
2nd Department of Gynecology and Obstetrics
University of Vienna
Spitalgasse 23
A-1090 Vienna
AUSTRIA

A. TACHIBANA
2nd Department of Gynecology and Obstetrics
School of Medicine
Toho University
Ohashi Hospital
2-17-6 Ohadhi, Meguro
Tokyo
JAPAN

A. TAHA
Department of Physiology
Faculty of Veterinary Medicine
Zagazig University
Zagazig
EGYPT

K. TAKEMORI
Department of Gynecology and Obstetrics
Faculty of Medicine
Kyoto University
54 Shogoin Kawahara-cho
Sakyo-ku, Kyoto
606 JAPAN

T. TAKESHIMA
4th Research Division
Imamichi Institute for Animal Reproduction
1103 Fukaya, Dejima-mura
Niiharugun, Ibaraki
JAPAN 300-01

F. TANAKA
Obstetrics and Gynecology
Osaka University Medical School
1-1-50 Fukushima, Fukushimaku
Osaka 553
JAPAN

M. TANAKA
Department of Chemistry
Nippon Medical School
2-297-2 Kosugi-cho
Nakahara-ku, Kawasaki
JAPAN 211

S. TANAKA
Department of Obstetrics and Gynecology
Sapporo Medical College
South 1, West 16
Chuo Ku, Sapporo
Hokkaido
JAPAN

N.T. TEA
Fondation de Recherche en Hormonologie
26 Boulevard Brune
75014 Paris
FRANCE

A. TENHUNEN
I Department of Obstetrics and Gynecology
Helsinki University Central Hospital
Haartmanink 3
00290 Hensinki 29
FINLAND

H.-R. TINNEBERG
Universitäts-Frauenklinik
Michaelis Hebammenlehranstalt
Hegewishstrasse 4
D-2300 Kiel 1
WEST GERMANY

E. TÖPFER-PETERSEN
Andrology Unit
Department of Dermatology
University of Munich
Frauenlobstrasse 9-11
D-800 München 2
WEST GERMANY

S. TROTNOW
Universitäts-Frauenklinik Erlangen
Universitätsstrasse 21-23
D-8520 Erlangen
WEST GERMANY

Y. TSUNODA
3rd Department of Reproduction
National Institute of Animal Industry
PO Box 5, 2 Ikenodai
Kukizaki, Inashiki
Ibaraki 305
JAPAN

O. TSUTSUMI
Department of Obstetrics and Gynecology
Faculty of Medicine
University of Tokyo
7-3-1 Hongo, Bunkyo-ku
Tokyo 113
JAPAN

S. UEHARA
Department of Obstetrics and Gynecology
Tohoku University School of Medicine
Seiryo-machi, Sendai 980
JAPAN

H. VAN DER VEN
Klinik für Frauenheilkunde und Geburtshilfe I und II der Medizinischen Hochschule Lübeck
Ratzeburger Allee 160
D-2400 Lübeck
WEST GERMANY

C.J.F. VAN NOORDEN
Laboratory for Histology and Cell Biology
University of Amsterdam
Academic Medical Center
Meibergdreef 15
1105 AZ Amsterdam
THE NETHERLANDS

L. VESELSKY
Department of Biochemistry
Institute of Molecular Genetics
Czechoslovak Academy of Science
Flemingovo nám. 2
166 10 Prague 6
CZECHOSLOVAKIA

P. WAGERBICHLER
1st University Clinic of Obstetrics and Gynecology
Spitalgasse 23
A-1090 Vienna
AUSTRIA

L.V. WAGEN KNECHT
Department of Urology
University of Hamburg
Martinistrasse
2000 Hamburg
WEST GERMANY

A.P. WALKER
Department of Obstetrics and Gynaecology
University of Birmingham
Birmingham Maternity Hospital
Queen Elizabeth Medical Centre
Birmingham B15 2TG
UNITED KINGDOM

F.B.S. WEHAISH
Department of Physiology
Faculty of Veterinary Medicine
Zagazig University
Zagazig
EGYPT

P.C. WONG
Department of Obstetrics and Gynaecology
National University of Singapore
Kandang Kerbau Hospital
Hampshire Road
SINGAPORE 0821

T. YANO
Department of Obstetrics and Gynecology
Faculty of Medicine
University of Tokyo
7-3-1 Hongo, Bunkyo-ku
Tokyo 113
JAPAN

P. YLÖSTALO
II Department of Obstetrics and Gynecology
University Central Hospital
Helsinki University
Haartmanink 3
00290 Helsinki 29
FINLAND

Y. YOSHINO
Department of Biochemistry II
Nippon Medical School
1-1-5 Sendagi, Bunkyo-ku
Tokyo
JAPAN 113

L.J.D. ZANEVELD
Department of Obstetrics and Gynecology
Rush-Presbyterian-St Luke's Medical Center
1753 West Congress Parkway
Chicago, Illinois 60612
USA

Part I

The Human Follicle and Ovum

Part I

Section 1
Follicular Biochemistry

1
Polypeptide patterns of follicular fluid at different stages of follicular maturation

J. HUBER, H. KARLIC, P. HUSSLEIN, W. KNOGLER, E. KUBISTA, P. WAGENBICHLER and W. SCHNEIDER

INTRODUCTION

The fact that some oocytes may remain up to four decades in the dictyate stage of the first meiotic division impressively underlines the biological potency of meiotic inhibition and promotion. Previous observations that resumption of meiosis in explanted oocytes can be inhibited by addition of immature follicular fluid *in vitro*[1] prompted us to investigate changes in follicular-fluid proteins and peptides during oocyte maturation *in vivo*, since we speculated that such changes might be entailed in meiotic regulation.

MATERIAL AND METHODS

'Mature' follicular fluid was obtained by follicle puncture from five patients who participated in our *in vitro* fertilization programme. Follicular maturation had been stimulated by clomiphene from day 5 to day 9 and administration of 5000 IU hCG as soon as the oestradiol plasma concentration started to decrease. Laparoscopy was carried out 36 hours after hCG application by standard techniques.The second group of patients consisted of four women in the fertile age, who were regularly ovulating. From these women 'immature' follicular fluid was collected in the course of gynaecological surgery during the first 2 weeks of their mentrual cycle. Immediately after isolation and puncture of the oocyte, follicular fluid was centrifuged; the cell-free supernatant was pipetted off and deep frozen at −20°C. Two-dimensional electrophoresis was performed by isoelectric focussing in the first dimension and separation on 18% polyacrylamide-slab gels in the second dimension. After electrophoresis, silver staining of the gels was performed as described by Merril, *et al.* [2].

RESULTS

Figure 1 shows the protein and peptide pattern of immature follicular fluid after two-dimensional separation and silver staining. An analogue separation of mature follicular proteins using the same amount of fluid is demonstrated in Figure 2. Since the patterns were almost identical within the two groups (four and five patients, respectively) it was possible to establish tentative 'standard maps' of mature and immature follicular fluid (Figures 1(b) and 2(b)). The most prominent difference in the protein patterns between immature and mature follicular fluid is seen in the molecular weight range of approximately 4000 daltons. In the two-dimensional gels of all four samples of immature fluid the same peptide could be detected as one distinct band (arrow in Figure 1). In two-dimensional separations of mature fluid isoelectric variants of peptides appear in the same molecular weight range (arrows in Figure 2). The most acid variant of these peptides, which apparently corresponds to the 4000 dalton peptide of immature fluid, is present in much lower concentration compared with immature fluid.

CONCLUSIONS

Although the major portion of follicular fluid appears to be a transudate of plasma there seems to be one remarkable exception: the relative amount of an acid 4000 dalton peptide (arrow in Figures 1 and 2) was reduced in mature follicular fluid while two small additional bands appear in the same region. We speculated that this peptide might be the 'meiotic inhibitory factor' and that inactivation of this peptide may entail modification to less acidic isoforms.

References

1. Tsafriri, A. and Charming, C. (1975). An inhibitory influence of granulosa cells and follicular fluid upon porcine oocyte meiosis *in vitro*. *Endocrinology*, **96**, 922
2. Merril, C.R., Switzer, R.C. and van Kevren, M.L. (1979). Trace polypeptides in cellular extracts and human body fluid detected by two-dimensional electrophoresis and a highly sensitive silver stain. *Proc. Natl. Acad. Sci. USA*, **76**, 4335

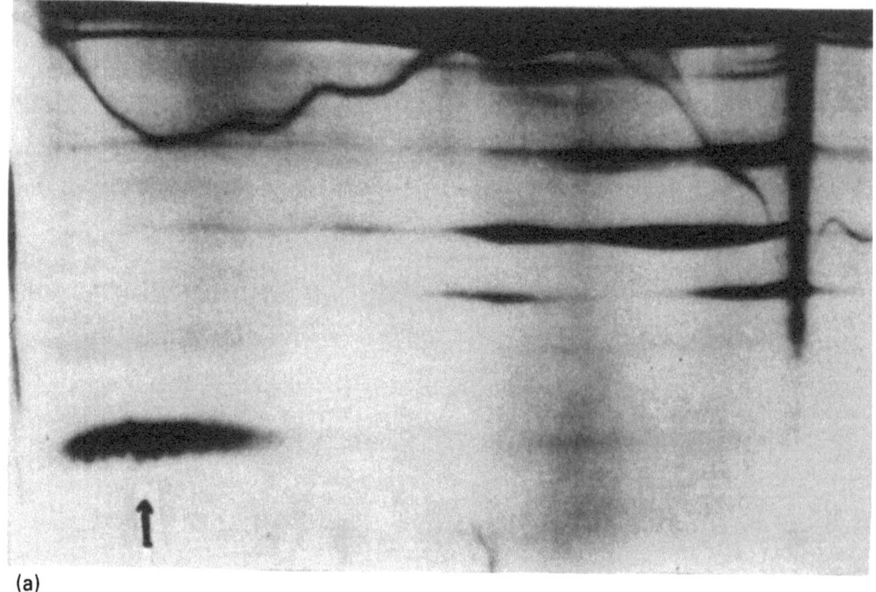
(a)

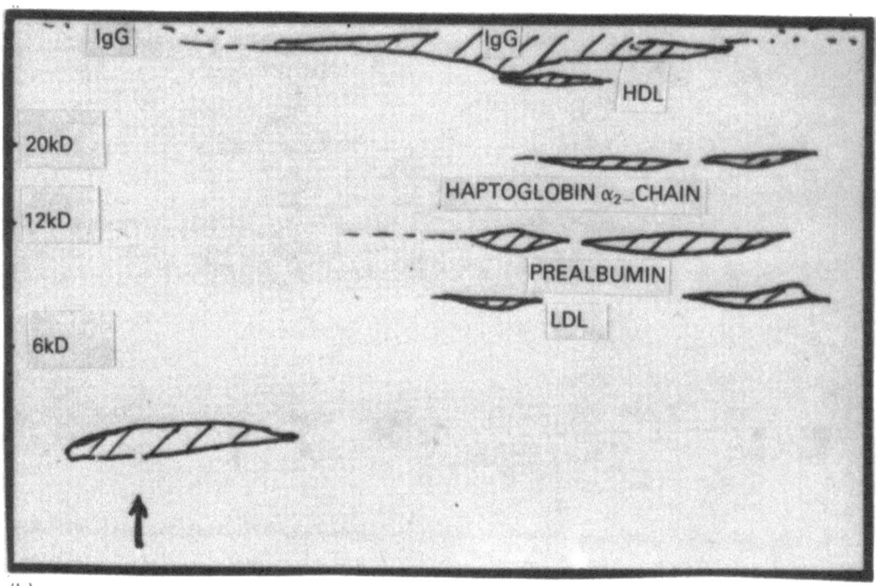

(b)

Figure 1 (a) Protein and peptide pattern of immature follicular fluid after two-dimensional separation and silver staining. (b) 'Standard map'

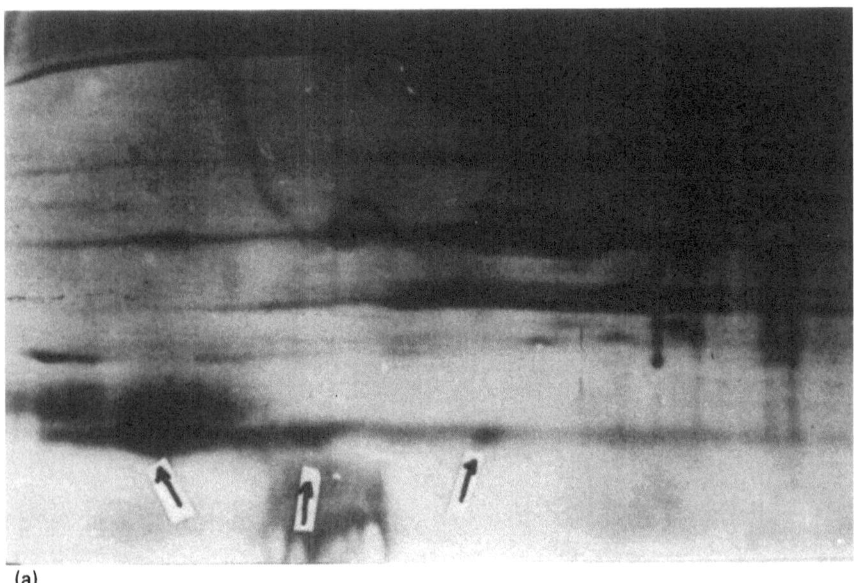

(a)

IgG Fight chains

20kD

12kD

6kD

(b)

Figure 2 (a) Protein and peptide pattern of mature follicular fluid after two-dimensional separation and silver staining. (b) 'Standard map'

2
Steroid hormones in human follicular fluid in assessing the biological characteristics of the oocyte

S. KURASAWA, S. SUZUKI, Y. ENDO, K. HATA and R. IIZUKA

The ovarian follicle has to be considered as a composite structure – namely oocyte, cumulus, granulosa, theca and antral fluid – whose components may exert regulatory influences upon each other. The maturation of oocyte is well correlated with follicular development, which consists of the development of granulosa on the theca cell layer and steroidogenesis[1,2].

When a follicle start to grow, its oocyte begins to enlarge and granulosa cells begin to multiply. In addition, it is known that the increasing diameter of the oocyte is associated with that of follicles, and most oocytes reach their maximum size after the follicular diameter reaches 1 mm.

In the present study, the concentration of steroid hormones in the human follicular fluid at various growing stages of the follicles were determined. Moreover, we assessed the morphological characteristics of the oocytes recovered from the follicles, and referred to the relationship between them.

MATERIALS AND METHODS

Each follicular fluid was aspirated from 124 follicles during operations for various gynaecological reasons or at the time of *in vitro* fertilization trials. Numbers of oocytes were recovered from aspirated fluid and assessed for their morphological characteristics.

After the oocyte was removed the follicular fluid was frozen at −40°C and taken for each steroid radioimmunoassay.

RESULTS AND DISCUSSION

The concentration of oestradiol in human follicular fluid is much higher than that in peripheral plasma[3]. The oestradiol level in large follicles was significantly higher than that in small ones and normal oocytes were recovered from oestradiol-dominant follicles (Figure 1).

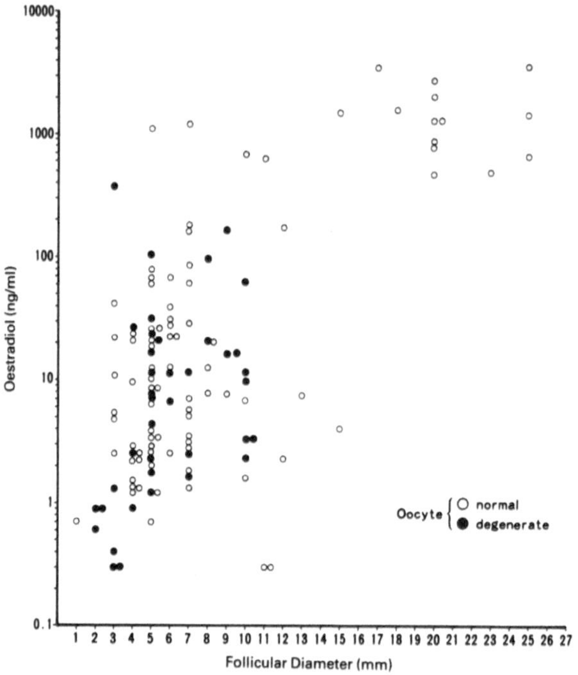

Figure 1 Concentration of oestradiol in follicular fluid

The concentration of progesterone was similar to that of oestradiol. Progesterone level in large follicles was much higher than that in small ones (Figure 2).

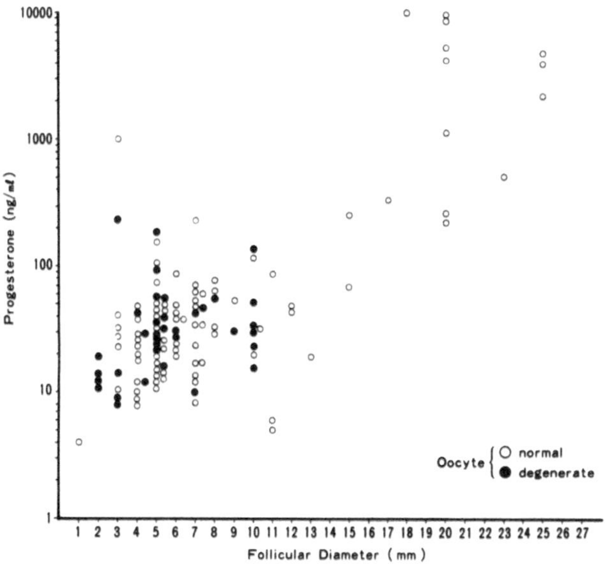

Figure 2 Concentration of progesterone in follicular fluid

The major androgen in follicular fluid is androstendione. The concentration of Δ^4-androstendione was not significantly different between large and small follicles, and atresia was not always associated with high follicular androgen level (Figure 3). In non-atretic follicles,

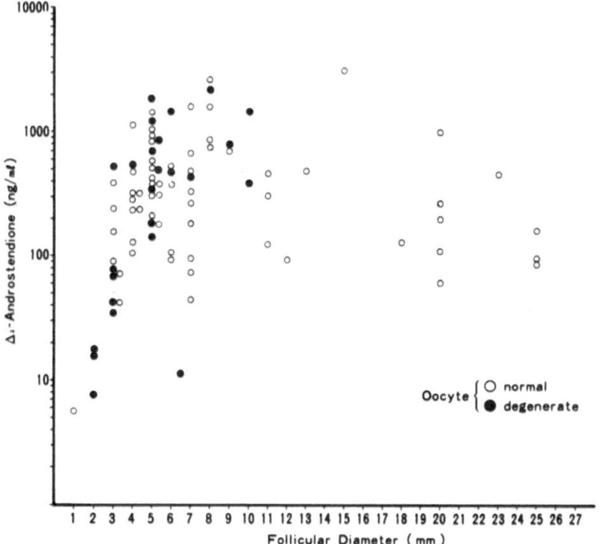

Figure 3 Concentration of Δ^4-androstendione in follicular fluid

androgen is well converted to oestrogen. However, during atresia, granulosa cells continue to synthesize Δ^4-androstendione, but the aromatase activity is substantially reduced and their capacity to synthesize oestrogen is diminished.

On the contrary, the concentration of testosterone in large follicles was somewhat lower than that in small ones. It could be said that concentration of testosterone in follicular fluid is gradually reduced as the follicle grows (Figure 4).

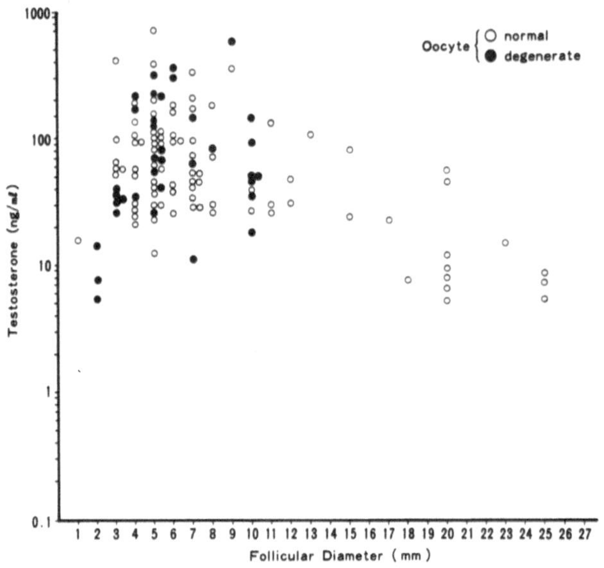

Figure 4 Concentration of testosterone in follicular fluid

In the group whose ratio of Δ^4-androstendione to oestradiol is high, the aromatization is poor and these follicles might be atretic ones. A high proportion of degenerated oocytes were recovered from these follicles. The ratio of Δ^4-androstendione to oestradiol of large follicles was quite low and we could recover normal oocytes from them (Figure 5). Decrease in follicular aromatase activity might represent an early event in atretic degeneration of antral follicles.

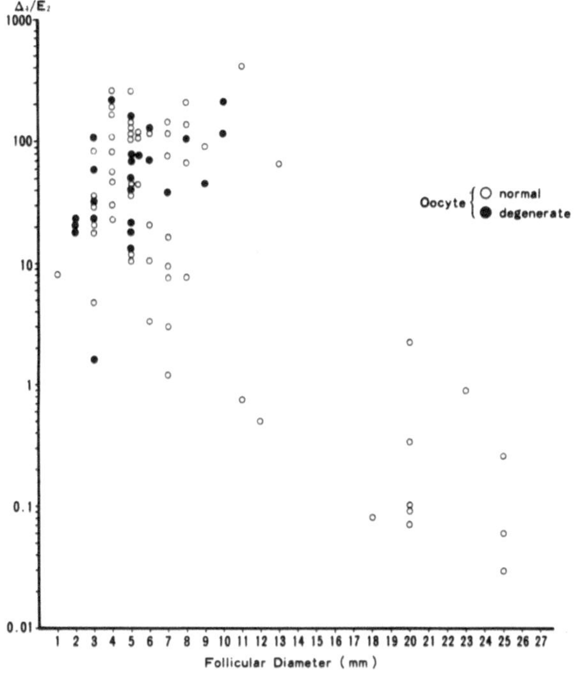

Figure 5 The ratio of Δ^4-androstendione to oestradiol (E_2)

References

1. Suzuki, S., Kitai, H. and Endo, Y. (1982). Morpho-functional characteristics of the human oocyte during maturation and fertilization. *Cong. Anom.*, **22**, 379
2. Suzuki, S., Kitai, H., Tojo, R., Fujiwara, T., Ohba, M. and Iizuka, R. (1981). Ultrastructure and some biological properties of human oocytes and granulosa cells cultured *in vitro. Fertil. Steril.*, **35**, 142
3. Suzuki, S. and Kobayashi, Y. (1977). Biochemical characterization of human follicular fluid. Presented at the *9th World Congress on Fertility and Sterility*, Miami

3
Concentrations of steroid hormones, prolactin and gonadotrophins in human peripheral venous plasma and follicular fluid

T. ENDOH, T. SATOH, S. TANAKA and M. HASHIMOTO

Follicular fluid is known to contain as many kinds of hormones as peripheral venous plasma, but few reports can be found on the measurement of six kinds of hormones. We measured concentrations of oestradiol-17β (E_2), progesterone (P), testosterone (T), prolactin (PRL), LH and FSH in follicular fluid and in peripheral venous plasma at various stages of the menstrual cycle.

MATERIALS AND METHODS

Follicles were obtained from the ovaries of 31 women undergoing various gynaecological operations. All of the women had regular menstrual cycles (25–32 days) and were considered to be endocrinologically normal. The stage of menstrual cycle was assessed from the presence or absence of a corpus luteum at operation, the pituitary and steroid hormones in plasma and BBT. The menstrual cycle was divided into three phases: the early follicular phase, the late follicular phase and the luteal phase. The follicles were classified as large ($\geq$ 8 mm) or small ($\leq$ 5 mm). Fluid and plasma were frozen at $-20°C$ until radioimmunoassay.

RESULTS AND DISCUSSION

The level of E_2 in large follicles ranged from 80 to 4800 ng ml^{-1} (n=19). At the late follicular phase, its level was apt to be very high ($\geqslant$ 1000 ng ml^{-1}). In small follicles the level of E_2 ranged from 1.0 to 1000 ng ml^{-1} (n=11). In all small follicles, however, with the exception of two cases, it was lower than 500 ng ml^{-1} at all stages of the cycle.

The concentration of P in large follicles ranged from 40 to 5000 ng ml^{-1} (n=20). At late follicular phase, some large follicles had a very high concentration of P ($\geqslant$ 1000 ng ml^{-1}). In all small follicles, the level of P was lower than 250 ng ml^{-1} at all stages of the cycle (n=11).

In large follicles, a correlation was observed between P and E_2 concentrations at late follicular phase (r=0.72; $p < 0.05$). It has been reported that granulosa cells acquire the ability to secrete progesterone at the late follicular phase *in vitro*[1,2]. In our study, some large follicles at late follicular phase were also observed to have lots of P and E_2. In small follicles no correlation was found.

The level of T in small follicles ranged from undetectable to 250 ng ml^{-1} during all stages of the menstrual cycle (n=8). In almost all of these follicles, however, it was higher than 50 ng ml^{-1} with the exception of one case. Thus some small follicles may have been atretic follicles since we took samples without histological examination. In all large follicles, the level of T was lower than 50 ng ml^{-1}. It is reported that the ratio of T:E_2 of follicles which have a high E_2 level is apt to be low[3,4]. In our study, a correlation was observed between E and T concentrations in large follicles ($r=-0.65$; $p < 0.01$), which correlates to some extent with previous reports. It is suggested that many large follicles were developing follicles at late follicular phase, based upon the high E_2 and P level and the low T level.

The level of PRL in large follicles ranged from undetectable to 80 ng ml^{-1} (n=13). In small follicles it ranged from undetectable to 110 ng ml^{-1}. The results showed no significant differences.

The LH concentration in large follicles ranged from undetectable to 75 mIU ml^{-1} (n=16); and from undetectable to 150 mIU ml^{-1} in small follicles (n=9). The FSH concentration ranged from undetectable to 36 mIU ml^{-1} in large follicles (n=8), and in small follicles from undetectable to 80 mIU ml^{-1} (n=8). Thus these results showed no significant differences.

We examined the relationship between the levels of hormones in follicular fluid and in peripheral venous plasma. The level of E_2 in follicular fluid at all stages of the cycle was between 20 and 100 000 times higher than that in peripheral plasma. A correlation was observed between the E_2 level in large follicles and that in plasma at late follicular phase (r=0.61; $p < 0.05$). It is speculated that E_2 was diffused or secreted from the large follicles to the peripheral plasma, especially at late follicular phase. Although a correlation was found between the P level and the E_2 level in large follicles at late follicular phase, no correlation was observed between the P level in large follicles and that in plasma. Therefore, it is speculated that a mechanism exists by which progesterone is prevented from diffusing from large follicles into peripheral plasma.

A correlation was found between the LH level in small follicles and that in plasma (r=0.68; $p < 0.01$). It is suggested that LH in plasma diffused into small follicles. However, the reason why no correlation was observed between LH in large follicles and that in plasma is not clear.

References

1. McNatty, K.P. and Sawers, R.S. (1975). Relationship between the endocrine environment with the graafian follicle and the subsequent rate of progesterone secretion by human granulosa cell *in vitro*. *J. Endocrinol.*, **66**, 391
2. McNatty, K.P. (1978). Cyclic changes in antral fluid hormone concentrations in humans. *Clin. Endocrinol.*, **7**, 577
3. Shoji, M., Kimura, E., Nakata, H., Ohkawa, K. and Hachiya, S. (1982). Relationship between morphological characteristics of follicular wall and steroid contents in follicular fluid during menstrual cycle. *Acta obstet. Gynecol. Jpn.*, **34**, 43
4. Brailly, S., Gougeon, A., Milgrom, E., Bomsel-Helmreich, O. and Papiernik, E. (1981). Androgens and progestins in the human ovarian follicle: differences in the evolution of pre-ovulatory, healthy nonovulatory, and atretic follicles. *J. Clin. Endocrinol.*, **53**, 128

4
Concentrations of steroids and prostaglandins in follicular fluids aspirated in an *in vitro* fertilization programme

F. LEHMANN, H.O. HOPPEN, CHR. SCHULZ, U. HAMERICH, S. AL-HASANI, H. VAN DER VEN, K. DIEDRICH and D. KREBS

Previous measurements of steroids in the fluid of human ovarian follicles have shown that follicles with high oestrogen concentrations (non-atretic) in natural cycles are the better source of oocytes capable of fertilization. Experiments with laboratory animals including primates have shown that prostaglandins (E_2 and $F_{2\alpha}$) are involved in the endocrine events leading to ovulation. Little information is available for humans so far. The aim of this study was to assess the concentrations of oestradiol, progesterone, $PGF_{2\alpha}$ and PGE_2 in human follicular fluid, aspirated after ovarian stimulation with clomiphene or clomiphene and hMG. Oestradiol, progesterone, $PGF_{2\alpha}$ and PGE_2 were measured in specific radioimmunoassays.

The therapeutic regimen included either 150 mg clomiphene from day 5 to day 9 or clomiphene in the same manner starting with 2 ampoules Pergonal from day 8 until the morning of the day when the hCG was administered. From July 1982 to February 1983, 78 women were treated with clomiphene and 52 women received clomiphene in combination with hMG. All women were given 5000 IU hCG when the leading follicle had reached a diameter of 18–20 mm; laparoscopy was performed 36 hours later. A total of 299 follicles were aspirated after clomiphene treatment, 286 after combined clomiphene/hMG treatment, respectively.

Table 1 Oestradiol concentration (in g ml^{-1}) in follicular fluid: relation to follicle size (ml) and method of follicular stimulation*

	Size									
	<2	2	3	4	5	6	7	8	9	≥10
Clomiphene:										
Total	96±93 (2–420) (*n*=18)	163±132 (6–186) (*n* = 15)	169±95 (30–365) (*n*=28)	153±85 (23–308) (*n*=20)	211±126 (15–402) (*n*=14)	140±76 (27–303) (*n*=14)	275±339 (5–1200) (*n*=16)	193±213 (46–1020) (*n*=17)	159±63 (33–270) (*n*=13)	112±51 (25–189) (*n*=19)
Transfer	–	328±100 (210–486) (*n*=4)	136±75 (38–246) (*n*=10)	143±72 (38–241) (*n*=7)	230±87 (65–322) (*n*=6)	132±97 (46–303) (*n*=5)	412±399 (35–1200) (*n*=9)	240±297 (81–1020) (*n*=9)	151±22 (134–177) (*n*=5)	92±57 (25–189) (*n*=7)
Clomiphene+hMG										
Total	81±90 (27–300) (*n*=8)	131±121 (13–318) (*n*=6)	205±205 (28–781) (*n*=18)	125±81 (65–355) (*n*=10)	258±283 (83–924) (*n*=8)	287±317 (34–1100) (*n*=12)	304±270 (85–826) (*n*=5)	353±305 (83–840) (*n*=5)	269±122 (99–376) (*n*=3)	175±190 (55–731) (*n*=13)
Transfer	–	240±71 (147–318) (*n*=3)	781 – (*n*=1)	94±6 (86–1012) (*n*=3)	100±15 (83–119) (*n*=3)	262±256 (116–827) (*n*=6)	223±71 (152–294) (*n*=2)	–	–	98±31 (55–155) (*n*=7)

★ Results are given as means ±SD, with ranges and number of subjects in parentheses.

Table 2 Progesterone concentration (in g ml^{-1}) in follicular fluid: relation to follicle size (ml) and method of follicular stimulation*

	Size									
	<2	*2*	*3*	*4*	*5*	*6*	*7*	*8*	*9*	*≥10*
Clomiphene:										
Total	555±465 (145–2100) (n=18)	920±500 (270–2080) (n=15)	1540±870 (165–3315) (n=28)	1255±895 (340–3650) (n=20)	2625±1675 (845–6900) (n=14)	1215±660 (415–3060) (n=14)	1240±1260 (120–5040) (n=16)	1190±450 (635–2190) (n=17)	2030±1725 (325–6670) (n=13)	1365±380 (690–2000) (n=19)
Transfer	–	1470±470 (790–2080) (n=4)	1480±1110 (350–3315) (n=10)	1345±925 (580–3650) (n=7)	1790±780 (960–3280) (n=6)	1140±230 (865–1560) (n=5)	1300±915 (540–3350) (n=9)	1065±455 (635–1870) (n=8)	1530±1150 (530–3690) (n=5)	1225±290 (935–1770) (n=7)
Clomiphene+hMG										
Total	1010±760 (560–2900) (n=8)	1355±890 (360–2660) (n=6)	1135±565 (420–2270) (n=18)	1445±750 (340–2830) (n=10)	1620±660 (750–3100) (n=8)	1175±635 (540–2900) (n=12)	1400±1050 (720–3460) (n=5)	1680±915 (340–3150) (n=5)	1535±230 (1210–1700) (n=3)	1095±575 (380–2320) (n=13)
Transfer	–	2080±710 (1080–2660) (n=3)	1560 – (n=1)	1800±740 (1145–2830) (n=3)	1155±205 (750–1380) (n=3)	1105±435 (610–1800) (n=6)	2125±1335 (790–3460) (n=2)	–	–	890±280 (56–1400) (n = 7)

★ Results are given as means ±SD, with ranges and number of subjects in parentheses.

Table 3 Prostaglandin concentration (in g ml^{-1}) in follicular fluid. Relation to follicular size (ml) and method of follicular stimulation*

	Size									
	<2	2	3	4	5	6	7	8	9	≥10
Clomiphene:										
Total	ND	4.0±3.0 (1.5–9.2) (*n*=4)	4.2±3.0 (1.7–9.7) (*n*=7)	7.7±2.8 (4.1–11.9) (*n*=5)	4.3±1.1 (3.3–5.2) (*n*=2)	4.7±1.8 (3.3–7.7) (*n*=4)	3.8±3.4 (0.9–12.8) (*n*=11)	6.5±4.3 (0.8–13.5) (*n*=5)	3.6±2.2 (1.3–7.6) (*n*=6)	3.9±3.0 (0.8–9.2) (*n*=5)
Transfer	ND	1.5 (*n*=1)	1.6±0.2 (1.4–1.7) (*n*=2)	8.7±0.3 (8.4–8.9) (*n*=2)	5.2 (*n*=1)	5.5±2.2 (3.3–7.7) (*n*=2)	5.1±4.2 (0.9–12.8) (*n*=6)	6.5±4.3 (0.8–13.5) (*n*=5)	4.6±2.5 (1.4–7.6) (*n*=3)	–
Clomiphene+hMG:										
Total	3.4±3.0 (1.4–9.4) (*n*=5)	2.7±1.0 (1.5–4.0) (*n*=5)	2.5±0.9 (0.9–4.3) (*n*=15)	3.9±2.6 (0.9–7.5) (*n*=5)	1.9±0.2 (1.7–2.3) (*n*=4)	3.7±3.1 (2.0–11.2) (*n*=7)	4.1±1.1 (3.0–5.1) (*n*=2)	2.2±0.5 (1.4–2.8) (*n*=4)	6.0 (*n*=1)	4.6±7.7 (0.7–26.2) (*n*=9)
Transfer	–	2.7±1.0 (1.5–4.0) (*n*=3)	1.8±0.9 (0.9–2.6) (*n*=2)	6.4 (*n*=1)	1.7±0.0 (1.7) (*n*=2)	2.3±0.2 (2.0–2.6) (*n*=2)	–	–	–	1.8±0.8 (0.7–2.9) (*n*=5)

★ Results are given as means ±SD, with ranges and number of subjects in parentheses. ND = Not done.

Table 4 Prostaglandin ($PGF_{2\alpha}$) concentration (in g ml^{-1}) in follicular fluid: relation to follicular size (ml) and method of follicular stimulation*

	Size									
	<2	*2*	*3*	*4*	*5*	*6*	*7*	*8*	*9*	*≥10*
Clomiphene:										
Total	ND	2.5±1.0 (1.9–4.3) (n=4)	2.4±1.8 (0.8–6.2) (n=7)	6.4±3.5 (2.2–11.0) (n=5)	3.2±0.3 (2.9–3.5) (n=2)	3.5±1.5 (1.6–5.8) (n=4)	2.6±2.0 (0.7–7.8) (n=11)	4.2±2.8 (1.2–9.0) (n=5)	3.0±1.8 (0.3–6.3) (n=6)	3.0±0.7 (1.9–3.4) (n=5)
Transfer	ND	2.2	1.5±0.7 (0.8–2.2) (n=2)	7.6±3.4 (4.4–11.0) (n=2)	2.9 (n=2)	3.7±2.1 (1.6–5.8) (n=2)	3.2±2.4 (1.1–7.8) (n=6)	4.2±2.8 (1.1–9.0) (n=5)	3.4±2.5 (0.3–6.3) (n=3)	–
Clomiphene+hMG										
Total	2.1±2.2 (0.6–6.5) (n = 5)	1.4±0.4 (0.8–2.0) (n=5)	1.5±0.3 (1.0–2.0) (n=15)	2.3±1.3 (1.1–4.7) (n=5)	1.3±0.1 (1.1–1.4) (n=4)	1.8±0.6 (1.3–3.2) (n=7)	3.5±0.9 (2.6–4.3) (n=2)	1.5±0.2 (1.2–1.8) (n=4)	1.3 (n=1)	2.5±2.5 (0.8–9.3) (n=9)
Transfer	–	1.5±0.2 (1.2–1.7) (n=3)	1.7±0.4 (1.3–2.0) (n=2)	2.8 (n=1)	1.2±0.1 (1.1–1.4) (n=2)	1.5±0.1 (1.5–1.6) (n=3)	–	–	–	1.4±0.4 (0.8–1.9) (n=5)

* Results are given as means ±SD, with ranges and number of subjects in parentheses.

When we noticed that we also had a reasonable fertilization rate with oocytes from very small follicles – and this was also true for clomiphene and clomiphene/hMG therapy – we became very interested in characterizing these follicles by the above-mentioned criteria.

RESULTS

The oestradiol levels as a mean increased with size and decreased again in follicles presenting with more than 9 ml fluid. It is important to note that even in very small follicles oestradiol concentrations can be very high. We found no real difference between the total and the value of follicles from which the oocytes could be fertilized and transferred. There was no difference between clomiphene and clomiphene/hMG stimulation (Table 1).

The mean values of the progesterone levels also increased with size but did not decrease in big follicles. No difference could be found either between the treatment groups nor between follicular fluids with oocytes leading or not leading to an embryo transfer (Table 2).

Prostaglandin concentrations can be presented as preliminary results in 106 follicular fluids. For the PGE_2 concentrations we did not find size-dependent values, although 4 ml follicles showed peak levels. Follicles in which oocytes were transferred tended to have higher PGE_2 concentrations than those that did not lead to fertilization and transfer. PGE_2 levels were found to be higher after clomiphene treatment than after the combined clomiphene/hMG therapy (Table 3).

$PGF_{2\alpha}$ levels were lower than the measured PGE_2 concentrations. Again 4 ml follicles showed the highest values. There was no difference between follicles in which oocytes were transferred and the mean values of the total group; also $PGF_{2\alpha}$ levels were found to be higher after clomiphene treatment than after combined clomiphene/hMG therapy (Table 4).

CONCLUSIONS

(1) *In vitro* fertilization can be achieved with apparently ripe oocytes also from small follicles.

(2) The endocrine environment of oocytes having passed through the first meiotic division can be the same in small and large follicles, although E_2 and P concentrations increased with follicle size.

(3) Steroid concentrations (E_2 and P) show no difference after clomiphene or clomiphene/hMG treatment in follicles of the same size when mean values are compared, but are high in small follicles which contained oocytes capable of fertilization.

(4) Prostaglandin concentrations (PGE_2 and $PGF_{2\alpha}$) show a clear difference after the two different therapy regimens. Values are higher after the less intensive clomiphene stimulation. There is no relation between the PG concentrations, the follicle size and the oocytes' capacity to be fertilized.

5
Prostaglandin $F_{2\alpha}$ levels in the human ovarian follicle

M.R.N. DARLING and L. MYATT

INTRODUCTION

There is now good evidence in many species to suggest that prostaglandins are involved in the series of events leading to ovulation. Le Maire *et al.*[1] showed that the levels of prostaglandin $F_{2\alpha}$ ($PGF_{2\alpha}$) increase before ovulation in the ovarian follicles of rabbits, and the synthesis of PGE_2 as well as $PGF_{2\alpha}$ *in vitro* has been shown by Sharma *et al.*[2] to increase markedly in the pre-ovulatory ovaries of guinea-pigs. Many workers including Armstrong and Grinwich[3], Behrman *et al.*[4], and Barbosa *et al.*[5], have shown that prostaglandin synthetase inhibitors such as indomethacin prevent gonadotrophin-induced ovulation in rats and rabbits as well as in primates.

Aksel *et al.*[6] demonstrated increased levels of $PGF_{2\alpha}$ in venous blood draining the human ovary containing the developing follicle when compared with the inactive side, and Edwards[7] reported higher concentrations of $PGF_{2\alpha}$ in fluid taken from preovulatory follicles than in fluid taken from three less mature follicles.

Similarly, Swanson *et al.*[8] demonstrated that the concentrations of $PGF_{2\alpha}$ found in human corpora lutea immediately after ovulation were significantly higher than in corpora lutea examined later during the luteal phase, indicating that follicular $PF_{2\alpha}$ concentrations were probably higher at the time of ovulation.

Finally, gonadotrophins have been shown by Plunkett *et al.*[9] to increase $PGF_{2\alpha}$ synthesis by human ovarian follicles in culture. Increased levels of $PGF_{2\alpha}$ within the ovary may increase ovarian motility or may weaken the follicle wall, by activation of protease or collagénase, as shown by Morales *et al.*[10]. Either of these mechanisms could be important in the process of ovum release.

It appears that in humans $PGF_{2\alpha}$ has a more obvious role in ovulation than PGE_2. This study describes $PGF_{2\alpha}$ levels measured in human follicular fluid during the pre- and post-ovulatory period.

MATERIALS AND METHODS

Follicular fluid was aspirated from 80 patients undergoing diagnostic laparoscopy as an investigation of primary or secondary infertility. Thirty-two specimens were discarded either because they were contaminated with blood or because the patient was thought to be anovulatory as determined by basal temperature charts, serum progesterone (< 20 nmol l^{-1}) and laparoscopic findings during the mid-luteal phase of the cycle. $PGF_{2\alpha}$ level was assayed in the remaining 48 specimens of follicular fluid using a radioimmunoassay procedure, described by Elder, and the results expressed as $PGF_{2\alpha}$ equivalents.

All patients, except four, gave a history of regular 28-day menstrual cycles, the four exceptions having regular cycles that were longer than 28 days. Dating from the onset of the next menses was not used as it was thought that this may have been influenced by laparoscopy and aspiration of the ovarian follicle.

RESULTS

The results of $PGF_{2\alpha}$ levels in human follicular fluid during the menstrual cycle are shown in Table 1.

DISCUSSION

The concentration of $PGF_{2\alpha}$ found in follicular fluid rises during the pre-ovulatory phase, reaches a peak at day 14 and falls after mid-cycle. Because our dating was by menstrual history, the exact timing of ovulation cannot always be certain, but despite some possible overlap of the day of ovulation between days 12 and 16, the mean level found on day 14 is significantly higher than those measured on days 12 and 13 and days 15 and 16 respectively. With two exceptions the levels of $PGF_{2\alpha}$ found in follicles aspirated between days 17 and 19 were low. These samples were usually taken from small cysts adjacent to a corpus luteum.

Five higher levels of $PGF_{2\alpha}$ were found during the mid-luteal phase.

Table 1 Prostaglandin $F_{2\alpha}$ ($PGF_{2\alpha}$) levels (in pg ml^{-1}) in human ovarian follicular fluid

Day	*5–8*	*9–11*	*12–13*	*14*	*15–16*	*17–19*	*20–22*
Samples	*7*	*6*	*6*	*9*	*7*	*7*	*6*
$PgF_{2\alpha}$	200	440	230	1250	850	420	420
	120	150	340	1500	250	40	90
	130	300	255	920	220	60	625
	440	187	620	1360	300	60	190
	378	320	460	600	460	60	110
	278	451	310	400	555	231	110
	208			584	307	108	
				615			
				557			
Mean	250	308	369	865	420	139	257

One of these patients had endometriosis and each of the other four patients had cystic ovaries, hence the availability of follicular fluid at this stage of the cycle, although a corpus luteum was present elsewhere on an ovarian surface.

Studies in rabbits, rhesus monkeys and rats have shown that ovulation induced by hMG–hCG stimulation can be blocked by the administration of indomethacin, a known inhibitor of prostaglandin synthetase. This block, however, can be overcome by the intra-follicular administration of $PGF_{2\alpha}$. Ovulation was similarly blocked by intra-follicular injection of specific $PGF_{2\alpha}$ antisera. In all of these reports the ova have been found to be retained within a normally luteinized follicle and despite indomethacin treatment, the preovulatory LH surge occurs normally.

We have found increased intra-follicular concentrations of $PGF_{2\alpha}$ leading up to ovulation which is consistent with the proposal that prostaglandins play a role at the follicular level in the process of ovulation. Accumulation of $PGF_{2\alpha}$ could be due to an increase in synthesis, an increase in storage or a decrease in degradation. However, in view of the effect of indomethacin an increase in synthesis is a likely explanation.

The increasing concentrations of $PGF_{2\alpha}$ found in follicular fluid leading up to ovulation with a rapid decline after ovulation is further evidence to suggest that locally available $PGF_{2\alpha}$ is a prerequisite for the mechanical component of the ovulatory process.

References

1. Le Maire, W.J., Yang, N.S.T., Behrman, H.H. and Marsh, J.M. (1973). Preovulatory changes in the concentrations of prostaglandin in rabbit graafian follicles. *Prostaglandins*, **3**, 367
2. Sharma, S.C., Wilson, C.W.M. and Pugh, D.M. (1976). *In vitro* production of prostaglandins E and F by the guinea pig ovarian tissue. *Prostaglandins*, **11**, 555
3. Armstrong, D.T. and Grinwich, D.L. (1972). Blockade of spontaneous and LH induced ovulation in rats by indomethacin an inhibitor of prostaglandin biosynthesis. *Prostaglandins*, **1**, 27
4. Behrman, H.R., Orczyk, G.P. and Greep, R.O. (1972). Effect of synthetic gonadotrophin releasing hormone on ovulation blockade by aspirin and indomethacin. *Prostaglandins*, **1**, 245
5. Barbosa, I., Maia, H., Lopes, T., Elder, M.G. and Coutinho, E.M. (1979). Effect of indomethacin on prostaglandin and steroid synthesis by the marmoset ovary *in vitro*. *Int. J. Fertil.*, **24**, 37
6. Aksel, S., Shromberg, D.W. and Hammond, C.B. (1977). Prostaglandin $F_{2\alpha}$ production by the human ovary. *Obstet. Gynaecol.*, **50**, 347
7. Edwards, R.G. (1973). Studies on human conception. *Am. J. Obstet. Gynecol.*, **117**, 587
8. Swanson, I.A., McNatty, K.P. and Baird, D.T. (1977). Concentration of prostaglandin $F_{2\alpha}$ and steroids in the human corpus luteum. *J. Endocrinol.*, **73**, 115
9. Plunkett, E.R., Moon, Y.S., Zamecknik, J. and Armstrong, D.T. (1975). Preliminary evidence of a role for prostaglandin F in human follicular function. *Am. J. Obstet, Gynecol.*, **123**, 391
10. Morales, T.I., Woessner, J.F., Howell, D.S., Marsh, J.M. and Le Maire, W.J. (1978). A microassay for the direct demonstration of collagenlytic activity in graafian follicles of the rat. *Biochem. Biophys. Acta*, **524**, 428

Part I

Section 2
The Granulosa Cell

6
The human granulosa cell changes during luteogenesis veiwed by scanning and transmission electron microscopy

S. MAKABE, Y. KANEKO, E. KOJIMA, G. OMURA and K. MOMOSE

The ultrastructure of human granulosa cells differentiating in lutein cells has been studied in an attempt to correlate morphological features with functional events. To date, the relationship between fine surface structure and interior cytoplasmic organelles has not yet been clearly explained.

MATERIALS AND METHODS

The ovarian samples were taken from normal and anovulatory patients (induced ovulation by hMG–hCG) ranging in age from 23 to 38 years. Patients were evaluated through an endocrinological profile. The granulosa cells were taken from preovulatory follicles.

The granulosa–lutein cells were obtained from corpus haemorrhagicum and corpus luteum at daily intervals to study their continued transformation under the influence of gonadotrophins. Ovarian samples were divided into two groups. All the segments were fixed in 2.5% glutaraldehyde. For SEM, the tissues were processed by critical point drying, sputter coated with platinum and palladium, and some samples were also made by styrene fracture and viewed by Hitachi S-450. For

TEM, samples were post-fixed in 1% osmium tetroxide, dehydrated, stained with uranyl acetate and lead citrate and examined by Hitachi H-600.

RESULTS AND DISCUSSION

In normally growing follicles (medium, large, preovulatory) the granulosa layer exhibits polymorphic shapes, which generally parallel the stages of follicular and metabolic activity. In the granulosa cells of maturing follicles, several surface evaginations – slender microvilli, ruffles, blebs and amoeboid projections – are observed in differing concentrations according to the changing role of the luteofollicular complex[1,2].

In atretic follicles, granulosa cells are of irregular size and shape, exhibit a few distorted microvilli and cytoplasmic extensions, and some appear flattened.

The role that cytoplasmic organelles play in the granulosa–lutein cell function has been determined. Mitochondria with tubulovesicular cristae are characteristic of steroid-secreting cells and contain the enzymes necessary for cholesterol side-chain cleavage. During the early stages of lutein cell differentiation endoplasmic reticulum increase in total amount, concomitant with a shift from rough morphology to a predominantly smooth reticulum during luteinization. Lipid droplets are considered to represent the storage site for cholesterol and for other steroid precursors or final secretory products[3]. The fine surface of immature granulosa–lutein cells obtained from preovulatory follicles exhibit numerous microvilli which have partially disappeared, while blebbing activity and pits (pinocytotic vesicles) become prominent. Many cells become irregular in shape and enlarged inside of these cells mitochondria with both lamelliform and tubular cristae, and rough and smooth endoplasmic reticulum and dense lipid droplets start to become evident. These cellular organelles suggest that initial luteinization occurs before ovulation (Figures 1–4).

In contrast, the surface of mature granulosa–lutein cells show a few microvillous projections and some blebs and many amoeboid cytoplasmic extensions. The cells become progressively enlarged, and of irregular amoeboidal shape.

Such surface alterations are accompanied by cytoplasmic changes, including appearance of abundant smooth endoplasmic reticulum membranes often closely associated with lipid droplets and mitochondria with tubular or villiform cristae. These aspects are related with increased steroidogenetic activity in the granulosa–lutein cells[4].

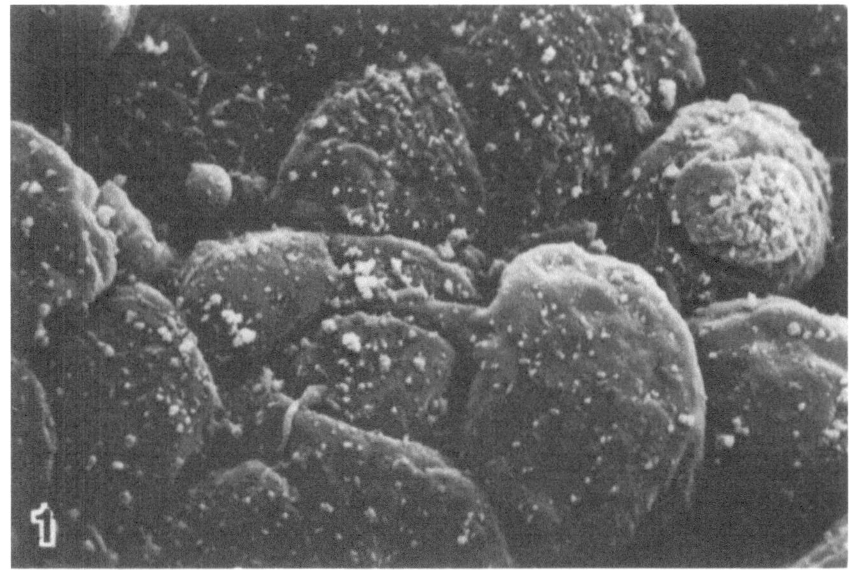

Figure 1

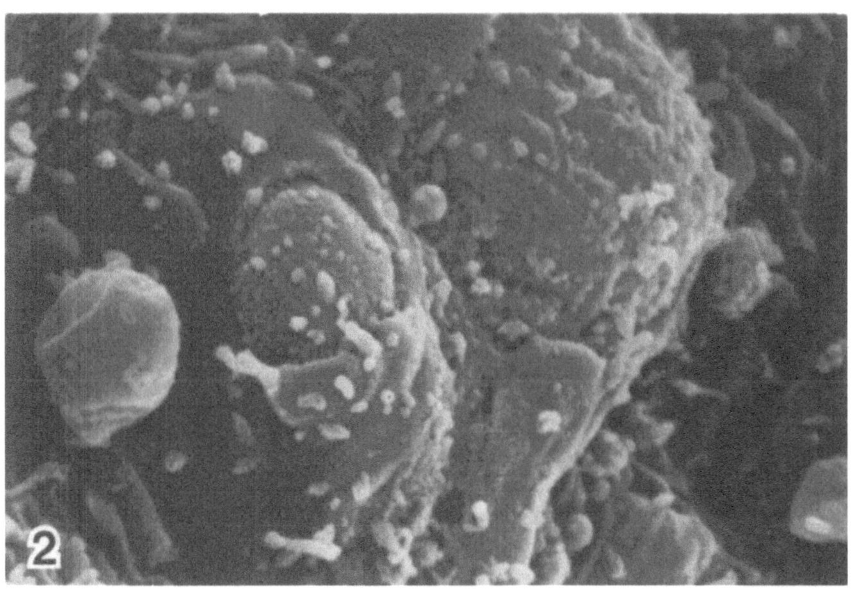

Figure 2

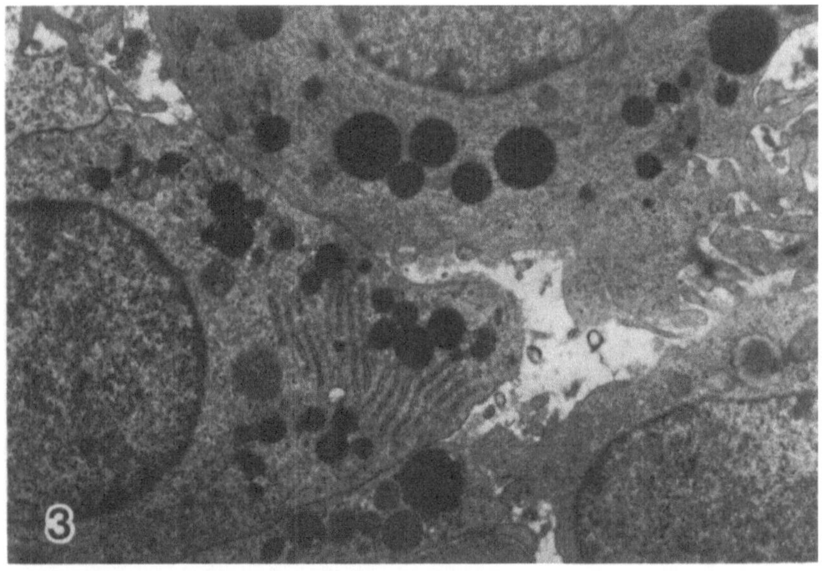

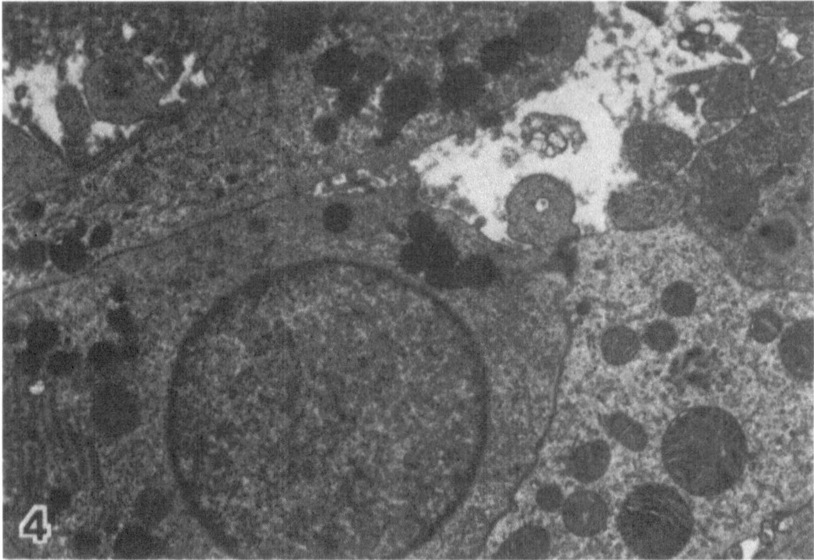

Figures 1–4 SEM and TEM of granulosa cells from preovulatory follicles suggest that initial steroidogenetic activity occurs before ovulation. (1) Note loss of microvilli and irregular shape. SEM, × 3000. (2) Note enlarged size and microvillous cytoplasmic extensions and blebs. SEM, × 6000. (3) Part of three adjacent granulosa cells. Note microvillous projections, lipid droplets, mitochondria with tubular cristae and stacks of rough endoplasmic reticulum. TEM, × 6000 (4) Note predominant blebbing, lipid droplets and mitochondria with tubular cristae. TEM, × 6000.

CONCLUDING REMARKS

In conclusion, our results obtained with correlative TEM and SEM samples of human granulosa–lutein cells demonstrate that the fine surface features of these elements are possibly associated with their steroido-genetic activity. Therefore, the surface profile of differentiating granulosa–lutein cells can be used as a good indication of their respective steroidogenetic status.

References

1. Motta, P. and Van Blerkon, J. (1979). Structure and ultrastructure of ovarian follicles. In Hafez, E.S.E. (ed.) *Human Ovulation*. pp. 17–38. (Amsterdam: Elsevier, North Holland)
2. Makabe, S. (1981). Scanning electron microscopy of normal and anovulatory human ovaries. In Didio, L.J.A., Motta, P.M. and Allen, D.J. (eds.) *Three Dimensional Microanatomy of Cells and Tissues Surfaces*. pp. 245–266. (Amsterdam: Elsevier, North Holland)
3. Nicosia, S.V. (1980). Cytological analysis of *in vivo* and *vitro* luteinization. In Tozzin, R.I., Reeves, G. and Pineda, R.L. (eds.) *Endocrine Physiopathology of the Ovary*. pp. 101–119. (Amsterdam: Elsevier, North-Holland Biomedical Press)
4. Makabe, S., Hafez, E.S.E. and Motta, P. (1982). The ovary and ovulation. In Hafez, E.S.E. and Keneman, P. (eds.) *Atlas of Human Reproduction by Scanning Electron Microscopy*. pp. 135–144. (Lancaster: MTP Press)

7
Morphological examination of granulosa cells in punctured follicles

V.MAAßEN, M.STAUBER, C. STADLER and H.SPEILMANN

Having established a reproductive biology laboratory unit in our clinic, we have performed an improved laparoscopic fertilization test in 69 patients. We decided to use ultrasonic measurement of follicle size and hormonal parameters. In 56 cases we punctured at least one follicle, finding a total of 73 oocytes.

We had difficulty in recognizing the exact quality and especially the maturity of the acquired oocytes, as have other groups which performed *in vitro* fertilization. It is vitally important at this stage to decide whether and how long the oocyte should be preincubated.

In one case, for example, we found two oocytes; one of these we classified as immature, the other as mature. Since the oocyte we classified as immature was later fertilized, we had to find other criteria to qualify the maturity of our material.

In this chapter we present different staining methods to disclose the condition of the punctured follicle.

RESULTS

The histological preparation of the follicle wall stained in haemotoxylin–eosin shows the functional change of the follicles.

When the granulosa cells of the follicle wall are closely packed and the thecal cell layer is poorly vascularized, we expect an oocyte *not* to be mature. When the granulosa cells are cloudy, sometimes desquamating, and when the thecal cell layer is much more vascularized we expect an oocyte to be mature. We found both morphological situations in follicles of 20 mm in diameter.

Granulosa cells within the follicle fluid were stained in orcein and Papanicolaou techniques. A distinction can be made between healthy (no pycnotic cells among the granulosa cells) and atretic follicles (pycnotic granulosa cells present). Number of cells undergoing mitosis and density of nuclei can be seen by these techniques.

During the transformation of the follicle granulosa cells into lutein cells, there is a gradual development of sudanophilic lipids to be interpreted as lipoprotein. The demonstration of this change gives a more exact picture of the follicle function. We use different staining methods to demonstrate this change. Each of these staining methods should not last longer than 20 minutes.

The quick staining methods used are:

i Papanicolaou;
ii Sudan iii, and
Sudan iii–Black B (air-dried smear)
iii Sudan iii, and
Sudan iii–Black B (frozen section).

We count the number of granulosa cells with sudan-positive areas, describe an approximate quantity of these areas within the granulosa cells (few, middle, much) and describe the way of distribution within the cytoplasm (small, middle or great granules).

CONCLUSION

We wanted to find out morphological criteria for the examination of punctured follicles. We are now able to differentiate:

(1) Mature preovulatory follicles.
(2) Immature follicles.
(3) Atretic follicles.

Cysts and hydrosalpinges which can be misinterpreted as a follicle should be excluded by morphological criteria.

Our aim for the future is to qualify the immature follicle by the different morphological techniques. For this we must find out how long we must preincubate the immature oocyte before fertilization can be done.

8
Development of ovarian follicles in readily ovulating patients during ovulation induction

S. LIUKKONEN, A.I. KOSKIMIES, A. TENHUNEN and P. YLÖSTALO

The growth of the human ovarian follicle both in natural and stimulated cycles has been studied in great detail by such illustrious scientists as Hackerlöer[1], Quenan[2], O'Herlihy[3] and Ylöstalo[4].

It has been established that the rate of growth in stimulated cycles is faster but the follicular diameter range at ovulation is similar to that during spontaneous cycles[3].

In this chapter we give our own results on the subject of follicular growth in cycles where several types of ovulation induction methods are used. In our *in vitro* fertilization programme we have had the opportunity to study the follicular growth in 100 cycles of 53 women suffering basically from tubal infertility. The patients' ages varied between 23 and 44 years with a mean age of 32.9 years. All patients had spontaneous ovulatory cycles before inclusion in the *in vitro* fertilization programme. A laparoscopy and ovum collection was performed in most of the cycles studied on cycle day 15. It was omitted only if ovulation had already occurred in the cycles where only one follicle had reached the diameter of 18 mm or more.

We used basically four methods of ovulation induction treatment which are presented in Table 1. We also performed laparoscopy and ovum pick-up in 15 natural cycles in which the follicular growth was monitored ultrasonically before laparoscopy. These cycles served as controls.

Table 1 Ovulation – induction methods

Clomiphene	100 mg daily,	cycle days 5–9.
Clomiphene	100 mg daily,	cycle days 5–9 + hCG, 5000 IU.
Clomiphene	100 mg daily,	cycle days 5–9:
plus hMG,	100–150 IU,	cycle days 10–13 (Group I).
plus hCG,	5000 IU,	cycle day 13.
Clomiphene,	100 mg daily,	cycle days 3–7,
plus hMG,	300 IU	cycle day 7 and 150 IU on cycle days 8–12 (Group II),
plus hCG,	5000 IU	on cycle day 13.

The ultrasonic monitoring of the ovaries was performed on cycle days 10–15 and in the case of clomiphene–hMG–hCG stimulation from cycle day 7 to 15. The number and the mean diameter of follicles were registered and the hormone treatment was adjusted accordingly.

The daily growth of the dominant follicle is presented in Table 2. The daily growth of 2.6 mm in natural cycles and 2.6–3.6 mm in stimulated cycles corresponds to the previously reported follicular growth rates. In the clomiphene-human postmenopausal gonadotrophin-induced cycles the growth rate is surprisingly slow, only 1.8–2.4 mm daily. However, the preovulatory diameter of these follicles is in range of the other stimulated cycles. A graphic presentation of the different rates of growth is given on Figure 1.

Table 2 Mean follicular growth (mm daily) during different treatments*

Treatment	*Dominant Follicle*	*Other Follicles*
No treatment	2.6(0–10)	2.0(0–7)
Clomiphene 100 mg	2.6(0.3–7)	2.7(1–11)
Clomiphene+hCG	3.6(1–11)	3.2(1–11.3)
Clomifen+hMG +hCG (Group I)	2.4(0–11.3)	2.5(0–7)
Clomiphene+hMG +hCG (Group II)	1.8(0–9)	1.7(0–7)

* Ranges are given in parentheses.

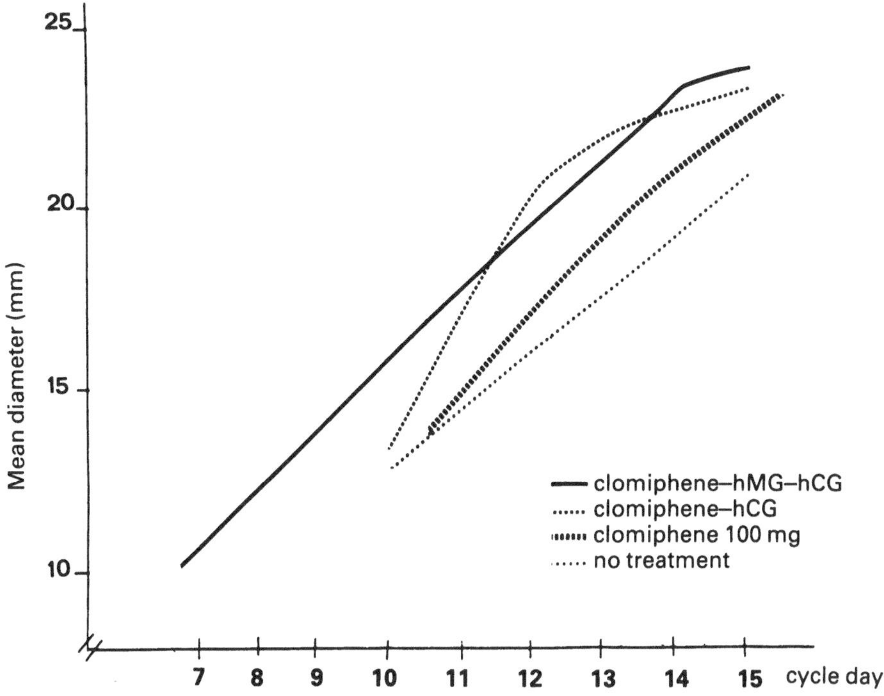

Figure 1 Mean diameter of dominant follicle during menstrual cycle for different treatments

The mean diameter of dominant follicle on cycle days 10, 13 and 14 is presented in Table 3. Even though the follicular growth rate in natural cycles corresponds to that in stimulated cycles the mean diameter of the dominant follicles is somewhat smaller on all the investigated cycle days. Unfortunately, our data is insufficient (only 15 cycles) to make definite conclusions. It seems that even though the rate of growth of follicles in clomiphene–hMG–hCG induced cycles is the slowest after cycle day 10, the diameter of the dominant follicle on cycle day 14, the day before laparoscopy and ovum pick-up, is the largest.

hCG was used in our series to enhance follicular maturation before laparoscopy and ovum collection, which were timed 36–38 hours after the administration of hCG 5000 IU. The effect of this amount of hCG was surprisingly that of slowing of the follicular growth, as seen in Table 4. The timing of the administration of the hCG and the discontinuation of other type of stimulation could also have affected the follicular growth at this point.

Table 3 Mean (±SE) diameter (mm) of dominant follicle during menstrual cycle

Treatment	*Cycle day*			
	8	10	13	14
No treatment	–	11.9±3.9	16.2±3.4	19.2±4.9
Clomiphene 100 mg	–	13.5±4.9	20.5±5.2	20.9±4.0
Clomiphene+hCG	–	13.5±5.0	22.1±3.4	22.1±4.5
Clomiphene+hMG +hCG (Group II)	12.8±3.6	17.3±3.6	21.5±2.3	23.6±3.9

Table 4 Mean follicular growth (mm daily) before and after hCG administration(5000 IU)*

Treatment	*Growth*	
	Before	*After*
Clomiphene+hCG:		
dominant follicle	3.8(1–11)	1.8(0.7–8)
other follicle	4.0(0–11)	0.4(0–7)
Clomiphene+hMG+hCG:		
dominant follicle	2.4(0–6)	2.0(0–8.3)
other follicle	1.8(0–6.7)	1.4(0–9.6)

* Ranges are shown in parentheses.

Table 5 Number of follicles detected, according to size and treatment

Treatment	*No. of Patients*	*Size (mm)* ≥7	≥15	≥18
No treatment	15	1.3(1–5)	1.2(1–2)	1.1(1–2)
Clomiphene 100 mg	25	2.3(1–4)	1.7(1–3)	1.5(1–3)
Clomiphene + hCG	8	2.6(1–4)	2.0(1–3)	1.4(1–3)
Clomiphene with hMG and hCG (Group I)	26	3.7(1–10)	2.9(1–8)	2.4(0–8)
Clomiphene with hMG and hCG (Group II)	26	6.5(3–11)	4.6(1–8)	3.0(1–5)

The number of follicles in each of the stimulation methods used in this study varied much according to what has been reported earlier on this subject. In natural cycles mostly only one follicle reached the diameter of ‹18 mm; in clomiphene only or clomiphene combined with hCG cycles 1.4–1.5 follicles reached this size. The best results were obtained in the clomiphene–hMG–hCG stimulated cycles where 2.4–3.0 follicles reached this size on cycle day 14, thus providing the possibility of three successful fertilizations in those cycles (Table 5).

Thus it seems that the group II type of clomiphene–hMG–hCG stimulation has the most obvious advantages in providing a larger number of follicles of larger sizes for ovum collection on cycle day 15. At present all our *in vitro* fertilization patients receive this kind of ovulation induction treatment.

References

1. Hackerlöer, B.J. and Robinson, H.P. (1978). Ultraschalldarstellung des Wachsenden Follikels und Corpus luteum im normalen physiologischen Zyklus. *Geburtshilfe Frauenheilkd*, **38**, 163
2. Quenan, J.T., O'Brien, G.D., Bains, L.M., Simpson, J., Collins, W.P. and Campbell, S. (1980). Ultrasound scanning of ovaries to detect ovulation in women. *Fertil. Steril.*, **34**, 99
3. O'Herlihy, C., De Crespigny, L.Ch., Lopata, A., Johnston, I., Hoult, I. and Robinson, H. (1980). Preovulatory follicular size; a comparison of ultrasound and laparoscopic measurements. *Fertil. Steril.*, **34**, 27
4 Ylöstalo, P., Lindqsen, P.G. and Nillius, S.T. (1981). Ultrasonic measurement of ovarian follicles, ovarian and uterine size during induction of ovulation with human gonadotropins. *Acta Endocrinol.*, **98**, 592

Part I

Section 3

Practical Aspects of Ovulation Stimulation and the Recovery of Oocytes

9
Endocrinological and ultrasonographic findings during ovulation

H. HOSHIAI, F. NAGAIKE, R. MORI, S. UEHARA, M. HIRANO and M. SUZUKI

One of the most important factors in establishing pregnancy after *in vitro* fertilization and embryo transfer (IVF and ET) is how to obtain a fully matured egg. We analysed endocrinological ultrasonographic findings during ovulation in two groups of patients, one with spontaneous cycles and another with induced cycles.

MATERIALS AND METHODS

Patients who had remained infertile for 50 menstrual cycles were submitted to laparoscopy for the purpose of collecting follicular oocytes in a programme of IVF and ET. In the spontaneous cycles, we retrospectively measured LH, FSH and oestradiol (E_2) levels in serum every 3 hours by radioimmunoassay to confirm the relation between the onset of LH surge and LH peak. In the patients with induced cycles, we prospectively performed ultrasonography and urinalysis of LH using Hi-gonavis and of urinary oestrogens using a new competitive haemagglutination inhibition reaction (Mochida Company, Japan). Clomiphene (Clomid) 100 mg daily was administered on days 5–9 of the menstrual cycle. From day 10 we began ultrasonographic examinations. When the maximum follicular diameter became 18–20 mm, measurement of urinary LH was started. When the onset of LH peak was detected before the maximum follicular diameter of 30 mm had been reached, we did laparoscopic egg collection at 26–28 hours after the onset. When the onset did not begin until after the maximum follicular diameter had been reached, we did laparoscopy at 36≃37 hours after the injection of 5000 IU hCG.

RESULTS

Serum LH, which increased 12–15 hours before its peak, increased rapidly 9 hours before the peak and then decreased suddenly within 9 hours. Serum FSH increased 12 hours before its peak, which coincided with the LH peak. Urinary LH showed almost the same pattern as serum LH. The onset of LH peak, confirmed by increasing urinary LH values, was 15 hours before the peak. The onset was defined by values over 50 IU l^{-1}. Almost all of E_2 concentrations in serum were more than 400 pg ml^{-1} through the ovulatory period in this study. But urinary oestrogen concentration measured with the new method revealed peaks before the urinary LH peak (Figure 1).

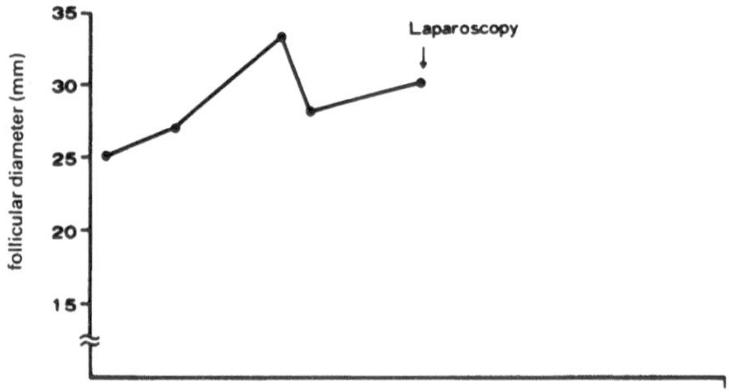

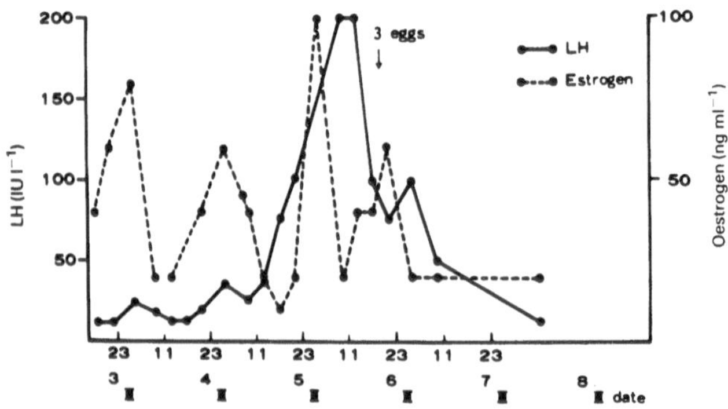

Figure 1 Time course of urinary LH, oestrogen and maximum follicular diameter in induced menstrual cycle with clomiphene (Clomid)

Ultrasonographic examination was done once a day before hospitalization and twice a day after that until egg collection. The maximum follicular diameter is increased gradually until ovulation, and at 20 hours before egg collection, follicular diameter was in the range 19–31 mm.

Egg recovery rate under laparoscopy on our IVF and ET programme was 72.9% per aspirated follicle and 80.0% per patient (Table 1). Finally, with this procedure we achieved two pregnancies following IVF and ET.

Table 1 Egg collection rate*

Year	*No. of patients*	*No. of follicles punctured*	*No. of eggs collected*	*Egg: follicle ratio(%)*	*No. (%) of patients with at least one egg*
1982	20	47	22(16)	46.8 22/47/	16(80)
1983	30	59	43(24)	72.9 43/59/	24(80)

* Trial egg collections were excluded.

DISCUSSION

Urinary LH measurement with Hi-gonavis is useful to determine the onset of LH peak, because urinary LH value is related to serum LH measured with RIA. Serum E_2 value may be useless because the peak value may be undetected with measurements of E_2 obtained every 3 or 4 hours. But urinary oestrogens measured by this new method may be helpful to confirm the onset of LH peak estimated by measurement of urinary LH, because peaks of urinary oestrogen could be always detected before the onset of LH peak. Additionally, this reagent has high specificity against oestrogen and gives results only 2 hours later. The maximum follicular diameters measured with ultrasonography are helpful but it is difficult to confirm the ovulation time because there are many individual differences.

We achieved five pregnancies following IVF and ET in 1983 which were induced with clomiphene (Clomid) and for which eggs were collected 28 hours after the onset of LH surge.

10
Laparoscopy for oocyte recovery

P. STEPTOE

Laparoscopy for oocyte recovery is carried out with certain modifications of the standard technique. At Bourn Hall, preliminary laparoscopies allow one to plan:

(1) The route of entry of needles, laparoscopes and ancillary instruments.
(2) The division of adhesions where the ovaries are found to be slightly involved, moderately involved or encapsulated. Mobilization of the ovaries or ovary is essential. Thermal coagulation techniques are always used for division of any adhesions except the slight avascular type which do not need haemostatis.
(3) The approach to the ovaries so that the difficulties of partial accessibility, which may still persist, can be overcome.
(4) To proceed to laparotomy

These have been performed at the Clinic with very reasonable success rates regarding subsequent *in vitro* fertilization and embryo replacement (Table 1).

Laparoscopy for oocyte recovery is performed using the special gas mixture 5% O_2, 5% CO_2, 90% nitrogen for the pneumoperitoneum. This is done to avoid exposing follicular fluid and aspirates and oocytes to high concentrations of carbon dioxide, which when mixed with body fluids will markedly affect the pH.

In order to overcome the possible risks of emphysema and embolism, induction of the pneumoperitoneum is carried out using carbon dioxide in minimal quantities. As soon as the needle is known to be in the abdominal cavity proper, then the CO_2 is switched off, and the induction continues with the 5:5:90 gas. A special modification of the gas apparatus allows this to be done very readily. At the end of the procedure the 5:5:90 gas is evacuated and replaced with approximately 2 l CO_2 which is then evacuated, thus 'washing out' any residual nitrogen gas.

Table 1 Laparotomies performed and pregnancies achieved at the Bourn Hall Clinic

Laparotomies	76
Laparoscopy for oocyte recovery	50
Successful OR and replacement	40 (80%)
Pregnancies	11 (22% of laparoscopies, 27.5% of replacements)
Abortions	2

OR = oocyte recovery.

OOCYTE RECOVERY

An avascular site is chosen for the introduction of an ancillary pair of forceps to hold or steady the ovary, usually about 8 cm from the midline on the right. A second pair of forceps holding a probing instrument is also sometimes introduced in a similar site on the left side in order to lift, hold or push aside any bowel or adhesion barring the approach to an ovary, particularly the left ovary.

Another ancillary opening is made with trocar and needle to accommodate a special double-channel aspirating/injection needle. This opening is usually near the midline low in the abdomen, depending on the planned approach to the ovary or ovaries. During the preovulatory phase of assessment, ultra-sound scanning enables one to see where the developing follicles are, that they are in an accessible ovary, and how they might be approached.

All openings are made with the assistance of angled laparoscopes transilluminating the abdominal wall with a high intensity of light.

The double-channel needle consists of a 1.2 mm diameter channel for aspiration of the follicle, and a 0.7 mm channel for the introduction of a heparinized culture medium into the follicle to wash out its contents and assist separation of an oocyte still attached to the follicular wall after the first aspiration.

The first aspirate in good folliculation is usually a clear, pale amber fluid which on microscopy may contain a few granulosa cells and viscous droplets. Sometimes the oocyte is found in the first aspirate. The suction used as a routine to start with is at 90 mmHg, controlled by a very accurate manually manipulated suction valve. The suction may be readily increased up to 120 mmHg. Thus the follicle is seen to collapse and empty as aspiration is performed. If the oocyte is not found in the first aspirate, the follicle is filled up with the culture medium and re-aspirated until the oocyte appears. The needle is kept in position until aspiration and washing is finished. Several washings may be necessary with long exposure of the follicle to the gas.

The timing of the laparoscopy (26 hours after the onset of the LH surge) usually is so good that mature oocytes are recovered. Occasionally at laparoscopy the manipulation may rupture a follicle, or rupture may have recently occurred. In many of these cases washing and suction of the operculum, adjacent ovarian surface and the follicular crater allows successful oocyte recovery, the oocyte still being held on the surface. Aspiration of fluid from the pouch of Douglas is seldom successful. All follicles of good size 2–4 cm in diameter are aspirated. The ideal ovarian response to superovulation is one where two or three follicles reach 2½–3 cm diameter in association with oestrogen increases of not more than 200 μg daily in urine.

After laparoscopy the patient rests for a few hours in bed and is ambulated early. Chest and shoulder pains are usually minimal and temporary.

Occasionally, laparoscopy has to be carried out before the 26 hour point (or 34 hours if the ovulation is induced by hCG injection). In these cases the oocyte can be brought to maturity by incubation *in vitro* using 1:1 follicular fluid and culture medium. Hence the value of obtaining clear follicular fluid whenever possible in the first aspirate. Large-diameter needles are not necessary and perhaps minimal disturbance of the follicles is the ideal technique.

11
A simplified approach to oocyte recovery for *in vitro* fertilization

D.J. LITTLE, P.D. BROMWICH, A.P. WALKER, A.M. MACKEN and J.R. NEWTON

While the effectiveness of *in vitro* fertilization is widely appreciated, its availability within the Health Service has remained limited due to the resources required. We describe our preliminary experience with a simplified approach. This relies on ultrasound alone to monitor treatment cycles and outpatient oocyte recovery by a modification of the ultrasound-guided transvesical technique described by Lenz[1].

PATIENTS, METHODS AND RESULTS

Nineteen patients were studied through a total of 37 cycles. The women were all slim volunteers and had been infertile for between 3 and 11 years. The infertility was considered to be unexplained in seven patients and in the remaining 12 couples related to absence of cervical mucus (5), oligozoospermia (4), endometriosis (2) and tubal blockage (1).

Ovulation was stimulated with clomiphene 100 mg daily from the first to the fifth day of the menstrual cycle. Daily ultrasound measurement of the mean follicular diameter was begun on the ninth day of the cycle. A small wheel mechanical sector scanner was used (ATL Mark III with a 3 mHz probe). When one or more follicles attained a mean diameter of 18 mm or more, 5000 IU human chorionic gonadotrophin (hCG, Profasi, Serono) was given intramuscularly. Oocyte recovery was attempted 35 hours later. The injections were given at 23.00 hours allowing the laboratory work to be completed within normal working hours.

Ultrasound examination before attempting recovery showed appearances suggesting that ovulation had already occurred in 14 of the 37 cycles. Under local anaesthesia a 19 cm 16-gauge needle was passed into the bladder and clamped to the ultrasound transducer thus ensuring that the aspirating needle lay in the plane of the ultrasound scan. The 16-gauge needle permitted the infusion of sterile warm saline into the bladder to optimize the degree of bladder distension. Under ultrasound visualization a 29 cm 19-gauge needle with a trocar pointed stilette (to fix the ovary during penetration) was passed into the follicle. The follicle was aspirated into a tissue culture tube then flushed with culture medium. Follicular aspiration was achieved in 18 of the 22 attempts; 11 oocytes were obtained from 10 women.

Most patients found the procedure uncomfortable, particularly the very full bladder. Analgesia was provided by Entenox (nitrous oxide) inhalation. The only complication was transient haematuria in four women.

Two of the 11 oocytes were immature, thus fertilization was attempted in nine; of these, two failed to fertilize; one underwent fertilization but did not cleave; and six were fertilized, cleaved and transferred.

Fertilization and embryo culture were carried out using a modification of the methods of Trounson *et al.*[3]. The embryo was placed near the uterine fundus using a Craft embryo transfer catheter (Rocket, London), the positioning being planned following a preliminary ultrasound scan.

DISCUSSION

The simplified methodology described avoids the need for operating theatre facilities, as required for laparoscopic recovery, and rapid hormone assays to time oocyte recovery. It might be argued that our low oocyte recovery rates (10 of 18 aspirations) and failure to achieve a pregnancy suggests that ultrasound timing alone results in less oocyte recoveries at the optimal point in follicular development. However, our results are similar to those achieved initially by groups using conventional methods[3]; we believe that our results will improve with experience. The use of higher doses of clomiphene will result in more follicles being available for aspiration in each cycle and would be expected to improve our results.

As anaesthesia is not required the number of cycles in which oocyte recovery is attempted may be increased giving individual couples a greater chance of becoming pregnant. Outpatient, unanaesthetized oocyte recovery and monitoring of follicular development appeared to help in reducing the stress caused by *in vitro* fertilization.

The double needle technique described has several advantages. The filling of the bladder can be optimized without requiring urethral catheterization. The aspirating needle passes through a sterile channel uncontaminated by the ultrasound couplant and cumbersome methods of shielding the unsterile ultrasound transducer are not required. The sheathing needle also reduces the flexion of the aspirating needle as it encounters resistance. Finally, the aspiration system was simply and cheaply produced within the Medical Physics Department. The transducer adapter and needle system are shown in Figure 1.

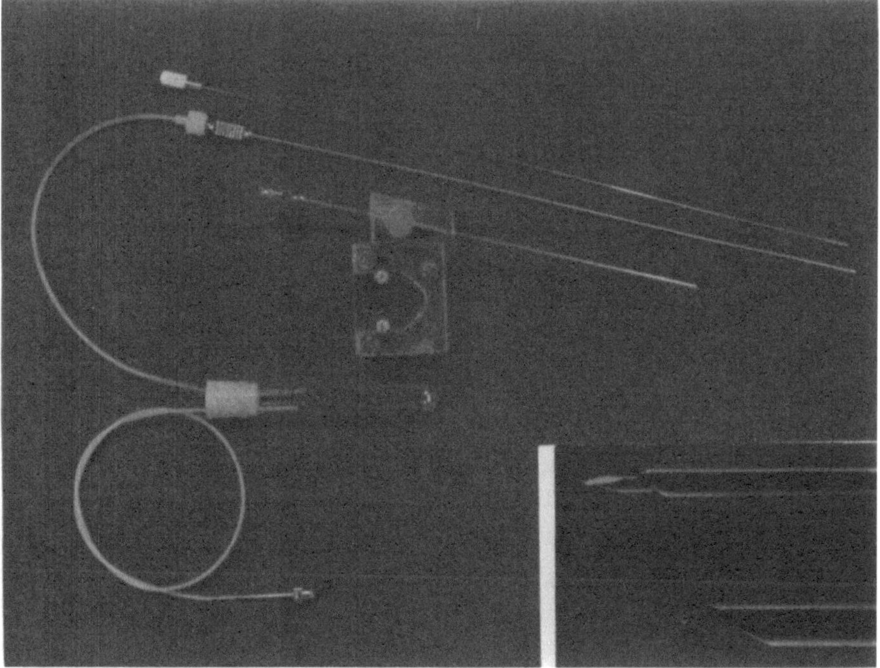

Figure 1 Aspiration system. The 16-gauge introducer is fixed in a slot in the Perspex attached to the ultrasound transducer fixing the needle within the scan plane. Inset: the modified needle tip (upper) developed from the standard chisel-pointed needle (lower) used initially

References

1. Trounson, A. and Conti, A. (1982). Research in human *in vitro* fertilisation and embryo transfer. *Br. Med. J.*, **285**, 244–247
2. Lenz, S., Lauritsen, J.G. and Kjellow, M. (1981). Collection of human oocytes for in-vitro fertilisation by ultrasonically guided follicular puncture. *Lancet*, **1**, 1163–1164
3. Mettler, L., Moritoshi, S., Baukloh, V. and Semm, K. (1982). Human ovum recovery via operative laparoscopy and *in vitro* fertilisation. *Fertil. Steril.*, **38**, 30–37

Part II

The Animal Follicle and Oocyte

Part II

Section 1

Biochemical Aspects of the Oocyte

12
Quantitative analysis of steroido-genesis in the single oocyte and pre-implantation embryo

O. TSUTSUMI, K. SATOH, T. YANO, O. ISHIHARA, K. KINO-SHITA, M. MIZUNO and S. SAKAMOTO

It is well known that fetal tissues, including the placenta, produce steroid hormones. The question at issue is when the biosynthetic pathway starts to work around implantation. Thus, an enzymatic microassay method was devised to determine the activity of 3β-hydroxysteroid dehydrogenase (3βHSD) in the oocyte and embryos.

MATERIALS AND METHODS

Preparation of the single oocyte and embryo

Immature oocytes with intact germinal vesicle (GV) were obtained by the puncture of growing follicles in the ICR mouse on the day of oestrus (day 0). Some of the oocytes denuded from the cumulus cells were cultured for 8 hours in the medium described by Biggers *et al.*[1] with or without 10 IU ml^{-1} of hCG (Mochida). Preimplantation embryos were obtained by flushing the reproductive tract on day 1–4 of pregnancy (day 1 = the day of finding the vaginal plug). The embryos were examined for developmental stage by stereomicroscopy. After freeze-drying, the oocytes and embryos were collected and weighed on a quartz fibre fish-pole balance[2] and applied for assay.

Assay procedure

NADH released by 3βHSD was amplified and measured as follows. 4 μl of the assay mixture consisted of 100 mmol l^{-1} Tris-HC1 buffer, pH 7.5; 1 mmol l^{-1} NAD; 400 μmol l^{-1} pregnenolone; 1 mmol l^{-1} EDTA; and 0.05% bovine serum albumin. A disposable plastic microtube (Eppendorf, Germany) was used as a test tube[3]. The reaction was started by adding the weighed oocyte to the mixture through the window opened in the wall of the tube. The microtube was tightly plugged with a Teflon rod to prevent evaporation. After 2 hours' incubation at 20°C, the reaction was arrested by adding NaOH to make the pH about 11 and the alkaline mixture was heated at 60°C for 30 minutes to destroy excess NAD. An aliquot of the mixture was added to 50 μl of NAD cycling reagent[4] and NADH in the aliquot was amplified 10 000 fold and determined fluorimetrically.

RESULTS AND DISCUSSION

Dry weights and 3βHSD activities of the samples in the developmental stages are shown in Table 1. There was no statistical difference among the dry weight on each day. 3βHSD activity was detectable in immature follicular oocyte and significantly elevated on the day of fertilization (day 1). The specific activities of 3βHSD increased from 51.9 ± 6.1 (day 0) to 84.0 ± 8.0 (day 4) nmol (mg dry weight)$^{-1}$ h^{-1} as they developed. This clearly demonstrated the presence of an enzyme involved in steroid biosynthesis, suggesting the production of steroid in the oocyte and early embroyos. 3bHSD has been detected histochemically in the preimplantation embryos of several species[5], whereas the production of progesterone from pregnenolone was not observed using radioimmunoassay or chromatographic analysis[6]. Therefore, some consider that the enzyme can be detected only after implantation[7]. The present result indicates that the ability of the oocyte to biosynthesize steroid hormones originates as early as in the follicular stage. The reason why the enzyme activity could not have been detected may be that the sensitivity of the methods used was not high enough.

Table 1 Dry weight and 3βHSD activity of mouse oocyte and embryos*

Day:	*0*	*1*	2	3	4
Stage	GV	1 cell	2 cell	Morula	Blastocyst
Dry weight(ng)	23.9±1.7	24.0± 2.3	23.0±2.2	24.3±2.3	25.2±0.8
Activity(pmol/h^{-1})	1.24±0.2	1.64±0.3	1.63±0.2	1.95±0.2	2.13±0.3

GV = Germinal vesicle.
* Dry weight and activity are given as means ± SD, (n=5).

The enzyme activity of the oocyte cultured with hCG for 8 hours (1.77 ± 0.05 pmol (oocyte)$^{-1}$ h^{-1}) was significantly higher ($p < 0.01$) than without hCG (1.34 ± 0.07 pmol (oocyte)$^{-1}$ h^{-1}). This suggests that hCG (luteinizing hormone) activates steroidogenesis in the oocyte. Progesterone produced in the oocyte may play important roles in oocyte maturation and development. In conclusion, the oocyte produces steroid hormone as early as in the preovulatory stage under the control of gonadotrophin and the enzyme activity increases during the preimplantation period proportional to the developmental stage of the embryo.

References

1. Biggers, J.D., Whitten, W.K. and Whittingham, D.S. (1971). The culture of mouse embryos *in vitro*. In Daniel, J.E. (ed.) *Methods in Mammalian Embryology*. pp. 85–116. (San Francisco: W.H. Freeman)
2. Lowry, O.H. and Passonneau, J.V. (1972). *A Flexible System of Enzymatic Analysis*. pp. 55–7 and 223–49. (New York: Academic Press)
3. Tsutsumi, O., Satoh, K., Sakamoto, S., Suzuki, Y. and Kato, T. (1982). Application of a galactosylceramidase microassay method to early prenatal diagnosis of Krabbe's disease. *Clin. Chim. Acta*, **125**, 265
4. Kato, T. and Lowey, O.H. (1973). Enzymatic cycling method for nicotinamide adenine dinucleotide with malic and alcohol dehydrogenase. *Anal. Biochem.*, **53**, 86
5. Dickmann, Z., Day, S.K. and Gupta, J.S. (1974). A new concept: control of early pregnancy by steroid hormones originating in the preimplantation embryo. *Vitam. Horm.*, **34**, 215
6. Bleau, G. (1982). Failure to detect 3β-hydroxysteroid oxydoreductase activity in the preimplantation rabbit embryo. *Steroid*, **37**, 121
7. Sherman, M.I. and Atienza, S.B. (1977). Production and metabolism of progestrone and androstenedione by cultured mouse blastocyst. *Biol. Reprod.*, **16**, 190

13
Enzyme cytochemical staining of isolated mouse oocytes with the use of a polyacrylamide carrier

C.J.F. VAN NOORDEN and G.G.DE SCHEPPER

INTRODUCTION

Determinations of enzyme activities in individual oocytes can be of utmost importance for the study of their metabolic processes. The biochemical determination of average enzyme activities per cell in homogenates has a limited value only, because oocytes obtained from an ovary can be in different stages of growth and maturation. Here lies the real value of quantitative cytochemistry, because the enzyme activity of each individual oocyte can be estimated. However, probably due to practical problems, enzyme cytochemistry has not been used often in studies of oocyte metabolism. The most common problems encountered are diffusion-dependent redistribution of coloured end-products over the cells in suspension, loss of oocytes during staining procedures and the difficulties of smearing these extraordinary large cells.

In this chapter, the use of a polyacrylamide gel as a carrier is described as a means of overcoming these practical problems with the cytochemical analysis of oocytes. With this new technique, the cells are incorporated in the gel before the cytochemical staining is carried out. This has been applied for the demonstration of glucose-6-phosphate dehydrogenase (G6PDH) activity with tetranitro-BT.

MATERIALS AND METHODS

Oocytes were obtained by repeatedly puncturing ovaries of 10–12 week old mice (Swiss random) in phosphate-buffered saline (PBS) with 0.1% polyvinylpyrrolidone (Merck, Darmstadt, BRD) using a 25-gauge needle. The cells were transferred to one drop of 100 mmol l^{-1} phosphate buffer (pH 7.0) at room temperature and washed three times in the same buffer. The cells were briefly fixed with 0.1% glutaraldehyde (Koch-Light, Colnbrook, Bucks, UK) in 100 mmol l^{-1} phosphate buffer (pH 7.0) for 5 minutes at 4°C. This treatment prevents bursting of the cells after they were mixed with the high osmotic acrylamide monomer solution[1]. The fixation is carried out in the presence of 20 mmol l^{-1} $NADP^+$ (Boehringer, Mannheim, BRD) in order to protect G6PDH activity against glutaraldehyde[1]. After fixation, the cells were washed three times in the same buffer.

Polyacrylamide films containing individual oocytes were prepared according to Van Noorden and Tas[2]. The procedure is shown schematically in Figure 1. The final monomeric mixture (160 μl) consisted of 50 μl of a buffered oocyte suspension, 100 μl of an aqueous solution of acrylamide monomers and 10 μl of an aqueous solution of riboflavin (0.004% w/v; Merck). The oocyte suspension contained 20 mmol l^{-1} $NADP^+$ for protection of the G6PDH activity during polymerization[1].

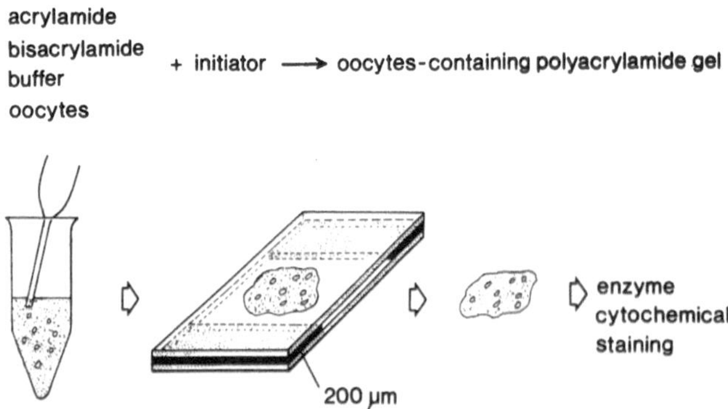

Figure 1 Schematic representation of the preparation of oocyte-containing polyacrylamide gel films

The aqueous solution (10 ml) of acrylamide monomers contained 1.92 g acrylamide (Serva, Heidelberg, BRD), 96 mg *N,N'* methylene*bis*acrylamide (Fluka, Buchs, Switzerland) and 121.4 mg Tris. The pH of the solution was adjusted to pH 7.1–7.3 with 5 NHCl. The polymerization was made to occur between glass plates with an intervening space of 195 μm. It was started immediately after mixing of the components and lasted 60 minutes at 4°C under ultraviolet radiation at 366 nm. The glass plates containing the polymerizing acrylamide mixture together with the oocytes were reversed every 5 minutes during polymerization to prevent these very large cells sedimenting on the surface of the lower glass plate and thus becoming only partially incorporated in the film and being lost[1]. After polymerization, the film was rinsed in 100 mmol l^{-1} phosphate buffer (pH 7.0) at 4°C (three times 10 minutes). Then the oocyte-containing film was dissected into a few pieces and incubated directly afterwards in the cytochemical medium for 10 minutes at 25°C. The medium consisted of 100 mmol l^{-1} phosphate buffer (pH 7.0), 4 mmol l^{-1} $MgCl_2$, 0.48 mmol l^{-1} $NADP^+$, 0.67 mmol l^{-1} glucose-6-phosphate (Serva), 0.1 mmol l^{-1} 1-methoxy-PMS (Dojindo Chem. Co., Kumamoto, Japan)[3], 2.6 mmol l^{-1} amytal (Serva), 5 mmol l^{-1} sodium azide and 1 mmol l^{-1} tetranitro-BT (Serva). Control experiments were carried out in the absence of substrate. After incubation, the reaction was stopped by rinsing the film pieces in 100 mmol l^{-1} phosphate buffer (pH 5.3) at 4°C overnight in order to stop the reaction and to remove unreduced tetranitro-BT. The film pieces containing stained oocytes can be kept for weeks at 4°C in this buffer without any noticeable change in the (tetranitro-BT)-formazan content of the cells. For microscopical observation the cell-containing film pieces were brought on a glass slide and mounted under a cover slip in a drop of buffer solution.

RESULTS

Figure 2(a) shows part of a polyacrylamide film incorporated with intact individual mouse oocytes after staining for G6PDH activity. The photomicrograph shows a well-preserved morphology of the oocytes and a sharp limitation of the formazan to the ooplasm. Figure 2(b) and (c) shows mouse oocytes after incorporation and staining for G6PDH activity in the presence and absence of substrate, respectively. It is shown that the formazan precipitation is restricted to the ooplasm, leaving the nuclear area and the zona pellucida virtually unstained. No formazan production occurs at all when the oocytes are incubated in the absence of substrate.

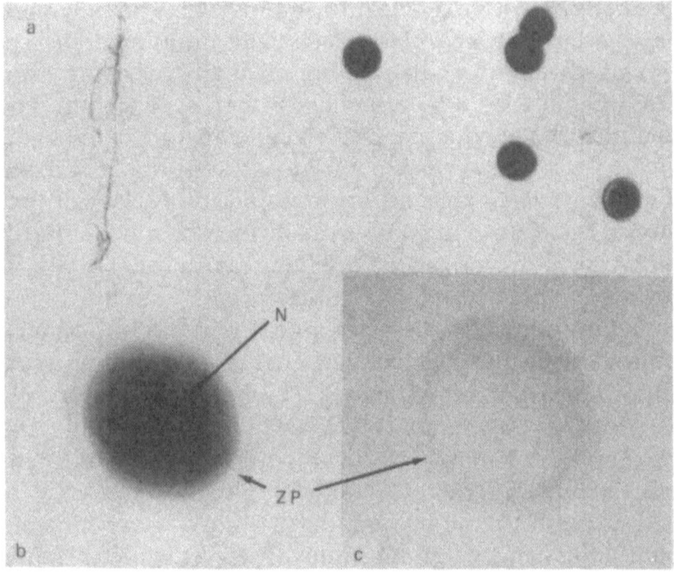

Figure 2(a) Photomicrograph of a piece of polyacrylamide gel film containing several isolated mouse oocytes and stained for glucose-6-phosphate dehydrogenase activity. (**b**) and (**c**) Higher magnifications of incorporated isolated mouse oocytes stained for glucose-6-phosphate dehydrogenase activity either in the presence of substrate (**b**) or in the absence of substrate (**c**). ZP = Zona pellucida; N = nuclear area. Magnification: (**a**), × 54; (**b**) and (**c**), × 195

DISCUSSION

Recently, we studied the possibilities of incorporating intact isolated rat hepatocytes in films of polyacrylamide gel in order to perform fundamental work on the cytochemical demonstration of G6PDH activity[2]. Because the incorporated cells kept a good morphology and the precipitation of the formazan produced occurred within the cytoplasm of the cells only, we decided to investigate the applicability of this incorporation technique for the enzyme cytochemistry of individual oocytes. From Figure 2 it can be concluded that the practical problems mentioned in the Introduction occurring with enzyme cytochemistry of individual oocytes can be solved when applying the new incorporation technique. A good morphology of the oocytes is maintained. Diffusion of either cytoplasmic enzyme molecules, intermediate products of the cytochemical staining reaction or the coloured end-product did not occur at all with these cells being incorporated in the meshes of the polyacrylamide matrix. Furthermore, loss of cells is completely overcome, which is of great importance for studying isolated oocytes. As far as we know, this is one of the first times that enzyme cytochemistry has been performed with consistent results on this cell.

The cellular formazan production can be measured with the use of a cytophotometer for obtaining quantitative data of enzyme activities per oocyte[4,5].

References

1. Van Noorden, C.J.F., Tas, J., Vogels, I.M.C. and De Schepper, G.G. (1982). A new method for the enzyme cytochemical staining of individual cells with the use of a polyacrylamide carrier. *Histochemistry*, **74**, 171
2. Van Noorden, C.J.F. and Tas, J. (1981). Model film studies in enzyme histochemistry with special reference to glucose-6-phosphate dehydrogenase. *Histochem. J.*, **13**, 187
3. Van Noorden, C.J.F. and Tas, J. (1982). Advantages of 1-methoxyPMS as an electron carrier in dehydrogenase cytochemistry. *Histochem. J.*, **14**, 837
4. De Schepper, G.G., Van Noorden, C.J.F. and James, J. (1984). Cytochemical determination of glucose-6-phosphate dehydrogenase activity in isolated mouse oocytes. *Acta Histochem. Suppl.* **29**, 149.
5. De Schepper, G.G., Van Noorden, C.J.F., Tas, J. and James, J. (1982). Cytochemical determination of glucose-6-phosphate dehydrogenase (G6PDH) activity in mouse oocytes with the use of a polyacrylamide carrier. *Cell Biol. Intern. Rep.*, **6**, 651

Part II

Section 2
Oocyte Maturation

14 Effects of A_{23187} and a calmodulin antagonist on maturation of guinea-pig oocyte

A. TACHIBANA, T. NAGAE, A. IWAKI, T. KINOSHITA, A. OKADA, K. NOKUBI and M. KATO

It is well known that oocytes of sea urchins and frogs resume meiosis upon exposure to Ca^{2+} and Mg^{2+}. The accelerating effects of Ca-ionophore on the maturation of oocytes have also been recognized. There are few reports, however, on its effects on the maturation of mammalian oocytes and the details are not known.

The purpose of the present study was to investigate the effects of A_{23187} and W-7, a calmodulin antagonist, on guinea-pig oocytes.

MATERIALS AND METHODS

The experimental animals were guinea-pigs weighing 250–300 g. Every morning, they were observed for the closure of the vagina, and then the ovary was separated from dioestrous animals under anaesthetic with nembutal. Isolated oocytes were extracted by puncturing the follicle in the culture medium. Oocytes or follicle-enclosed oocytes, which were removed from the ovary, were the subjects of the present study. The procedures of experiments are shown in Figure 1.

Follicle-enclosed oocytes were provided with isolated conditions. Cumulus cells were removed by adding 0.1% hyaluronidase to the solution and further removed by pipetting. The cumulus cell-free oocytes were fixed in alcohol acetate for about 24 hours and stained with

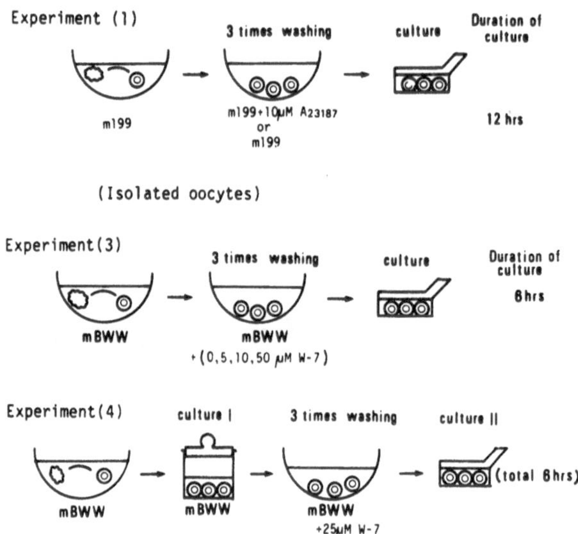

Figure 1 Experimental procedures to investigate effects of A_{23187} and W-7 on guinea-pig oocytes. Experiment 2, on follicle-enclosed oocytes, provided the oocytes with isolated conditions (at 37°C in air).
m199 = modified TC 199 by Yanagimachi[4]
mBWW = by Biggers *et al* 1971 (modified L-glutamine 20 ng ml^{-1} bovine serum albumin 3 mg ml^{-1})

orcein acetate. The maturation of the oocytes was classified according to the Donahue[1] report.

RESULTS

The effects of A_{23187} on isolated oocytes (Table 1)

When A_{23187} was added, the maturation of oocytes was: 20% at germinal vesicle, 47% reaching prometaphase, 18% reaching metaphase I, 9% reaching anaphase I and 7% degenerated. 74% of the oocytes matured to the phase of germinal vesicle breakdown or later. Maturation to metaphase I or later was observed in 27% of the oocytes, while in the control group it was as high as 77%. The inhibitory effects of A_{23187} are clearly seen.

The effects of A_{23187} on follicle-enclosed oocytes

No oocytes were at the germinal vesicle phase. 43% of the oocytes were at the germinal vesicle breakdown phase, with 14% at prometaphase,

Table 1 The effect of A_{23187} on isolated oocytes

A_{23187} (μmol l^{-1})	*No. of oocytes*	*G V (%)*	*Pro M (%)*	*M I (%)*	*Ana I (%)*	*Degenerated (%)*	*Maturing (%)*	*X(%) (X≥Meta)*
0	48	6(13)	5(10)	27(56)	10(21)	0	42(87)	37(77)
10	45	9(20)	21(47)	8(18)	4(9)	3(7)	33(74)	12(27)

G V = Germinal vesicle; Pro M = prometaphase; M I = metaphase I; Ana I = anaphase I; Meta = metaphase.

Table 2 The effect of A_{23187} on follicle–enclosed oocytes

A_{23187} (μmol l^{-1})	*No. of oocytes*	*G V (%)*	*GVBD (%)*	*Pro M (%)*	*M I (%)*	*Ana I (%)*	*Maturing (%)*	*X(%) (X≥Meta)*
0	13	2(15)	6(46)	4(31)	1(8)	0	11(85)	1(8)
10	14	0	6(43)	2(14)	4(29)	2(14)	14(100)	6(43)

GV = Germinal vesicle; GVBD = germinal vesicle breakdown; Pro M = prometaphase; MI = metaphase I; Ana I = anaphase; Meta = metaphase.

29% at metaphase I and 14% at anaphase I. In the experimental group 100% of the oocytes matured to the germinal vesicle breakdown phase or later, while in the control group 85% of the oocytes did. 43% of the oocytes were at metaphase I or higher compared with 8% of oocytes in the control group, indicating that the maturation processes were stimulated appreciably (Table 2).

The effects of W-7 (Table 3)

When W-7 was added, about 20% of oocytes were at the germinal vesicle phase compared with 7% of oocytes in the control group. In the W-7 added group, about 20–37% of oocytes inhibited germinal vesicle breakage compared with 7% of the oocytes in the control group. This indicates that the inhibitory effects of W-7 appeared early in the maturation process. When maturation progressed to the germinal vesicle breakage phase or later, half of the oocytes in the control group matured to the spindle formation stage or beyond. In contrast, the corresponding figures for the W-7 added groups were 19%, 7% and 13% respectively. Therefore, it was assumed that W-7 was active somewhere between the circularly arranged chromatin and spindle formation stages.

Table 3 The effects of W–7

W–7 ($\mu mol\ l^{-1}$)	*No. of oocytes*	*GV (%)*	*GVBD (%)*	*Con Ch–Cir Ch (%)*	*Spin–Meta I (%)*
0	31	2(7)	2(7)	13(42)	14(44)
5	16	3(19)	4(25)	6(36)	3(19)
10	30	6(20)	11(37)	11(36)	2(7)
50	15	3(20)	3(20)	7(47)	2(13)

GV = Germinal vesicle; GVBD = germinal vesicle breakdown; Con Ch = condensing chromatin; Cir Ch = circularly arranged chromatin; Spin = spindle formation; Spin–Meta I = spindle metaphase I.

Incubation of oocytes in medium containing W-7 after a 150-minute pre-culture (Table 4)

The spindle formation stage was seen in 4% of the oocytes in the W-7 added groups and 50% of oocytes in the control group. Again, W-7 had inhibitory effects on maturation.

Table 4 Effect of W–7 after culture I

W–7 (μmol l⁻¹)	*No. of oocytes*	*GV (%)*	*GVBD (%)*	*Con Ch–Cir Ch (%)*	*Spin–Meta I (%)*
0→0	24	0	6(25)	6(25)	12(50)
0→25	23	4(17)	10(44)	8(35)	1(4)

For list of abbreviations, see Table 3.

CONCLUSIONS

Our experiments with the cation A_{23187} on guinea-pig oocytes revealed that A_{23187} had inhibitory effects on maturation in the case of isolated oocytes as described by Jagiello *et al.*[2], while it had accelerating effects on maturation in the case of follicle-enclosed oocytes[3]. It was very interesting to observe that opposite results were obtained in oocytes of the same species of animal.

Follicle-enclosed oocytes have a follicular membrane in the follicular fluid. The mechanism of these as regards inhibiting maturation, however, is not known and requires further study.

References

1. Donahue, R.G. (1968). Maturation of the mouse oocyte *in vitro*. *J. Exp. Zool.*, **169**, 237–250
2. Jagiello, G., Ducayen, M.B., Downey, R. and Jonassen, A. (1982). Alterations of mammalian oocyte meiosis I with divalent cations and calmodulin. *Cell calcium*, **3**, 153–162
3. Tsafrir, A. and Bar-Ami, S. (1978). Role of divalent cations in the resumption of meiosis of rat oocytes. *J. Exp. Zool.*, **205**, 293–300
4. Yanagimachi, R. (1978). Calcium requirement for sperm-egg fusion in mammals. *Biol. Reprod.*, **19**, 949–1003

15
Effects of hCG, oestradiol and progesterone on mouse oocyte maturation *in vitro*

F. KAYAMA, M. MIZUNO, Y. MORITA, K. SATO and S. SAKAMOTO

There are many reports on the role of LH, oestrogen, progesterone, OMI, calcium ion and so on, in the mysterious process of oocyte maturation. In the majority of these studies, only nuclear change – namely germinal vesicle breakdown (GVB) – was employed as an indicator of the maturation. Although GVB is an important key phase of maturation, it in no way represents the whole process of maturation. Apart from GVB, little is known about the oocyte maturation resulting in sperm–egg fusion *per se*. In this report, the effects of hCG, oestradiol and progesterone on oocyte maturation will be described with special reference to the process acquiring fertilizability using the method of *in vitro* fertilization.

MATERIALS AND METHODS

Ovarian oocytes were collected from ovaries of mature Swiss albino female mice by puncturing with a fine needle. The animals were given 10 IU PMS 48 hours before they were killed. Oocytes with cumulus cells and without cumulus cells were cultured separately. Modified Krebs–Ringer solution developed by Toyoda *et al.* was used for collection and culture of oocytes. The oocytes were cultured in the medium containing hCG (2 IU ml^{-1}, 10 IU ml^{-1}), oestradiol (2 μg ml^{-1}) or progesterone

(2 μg ml^{-1}). Simple Toyoda's medium and Toyoda's medium containing DMSO were prepared for control groups. DMSO was used as a solvent of oestradiol and progesterone. Oocytes were cultured in each medium for 10 hours and then inseminated. Spermatozoa from cauda epididymis of male mice had been capacitated by incubating them for 2 hours before insemination. Observation was carried out under a phase-contrast microscope 1–2 hours after insemination. The oocytes were fixed and stained for further observation.

RESULTS

Effects of hCG – The frequency of GVB was about 80–90% in the control, 2 IU ml^{-1} hCG and 10 IU ml^{-1} hCG groups. hCG did not affect the incidence of GVB. The incidence of oocytes completing the first polar body formation was lower (5%) in hCG-treated groups than in the control (about 10%). Cumulus cells were observed to be detached from zona pellucida at a higher incidence in the 10 IU ml^{-1} hCG group than in the controls. 10 IU ml^{-1} hCG increased the incidence of oocytes penetrated by spermatozoa through zona pellucida in both cumulus-enclosed and cumulus-free oocytes. In cumulus-enclosed oocytes of the 10 IU ml^{-1} hCG group, a significantly higher incidence of sperm–egg fusion was observed than in the control and the 2 IU ml^{-1} hCG groups (Figure 1). In cumulus-free oocytes, 2 IU ml^{-1} hCG as well as 10 IU ml^{-1} hCG increased the incidence of fertilization, but not significantly.

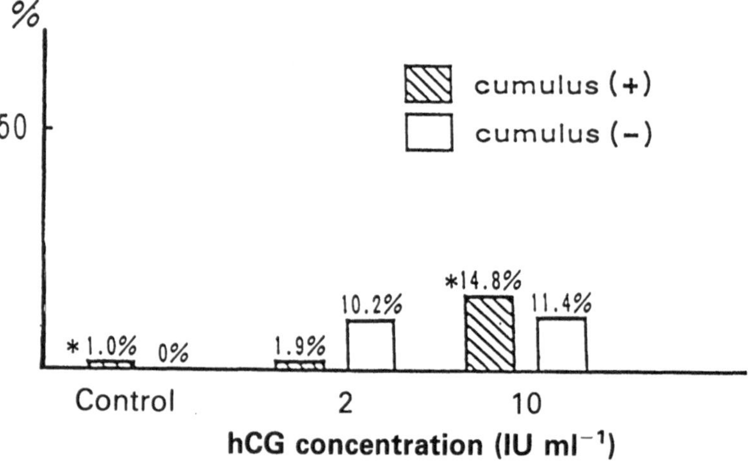

Figure 1 Effect of hCG on sperm–egg fusion.* Difference between values significantly different at $p < 0.01$

Effects of oestradiol and progesterone – The frequency of GVB was about 80–90% in the control (DMSO), oestradiol-treated and progesterone-treated groups without significant difference. The incidence on oocytes completing first polar body formation was low in each group. The incidence of oocytes with cumulus cells dispersed during incubation was almost the same between each group. No significant difference was observed between the incidence of oocytes penetrated by spermatozoa through zona pellucida in each group. Both in cumulus-enclosed and cumulus-free oocytes of progesterone-treated groups, a significantly higher rate of fertilization was observed than in the control and oestradiol-treated groups (Figure 2).

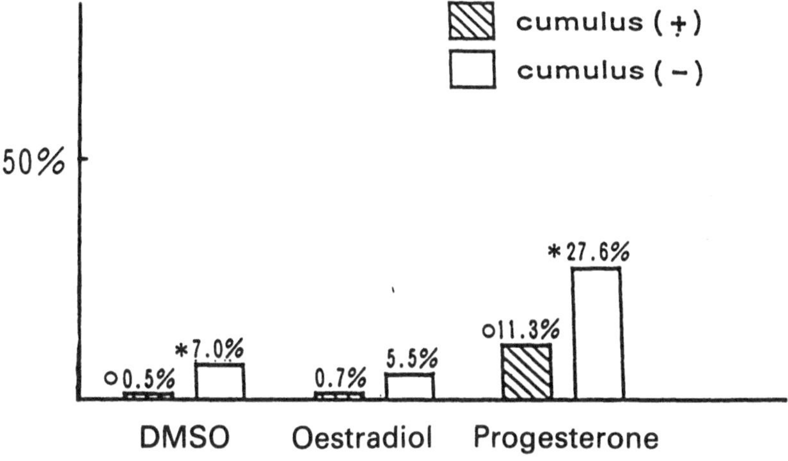

Figure 2 Effect of oestradiol (2 μg ml^{-1}) and progesterone (2 μg ml^{-1}) on sperm–egg fusion. o,* Difference between values significantly different at $p < 0.01$

DISCUSSION

GVB is known to occur by a simple releasing of oocytes from ovary. hCG, oestradiol and progesterone were suggested not to increase the incidence of GVB and polar body formation in this kind of experimental design. 10 IU ml^{-1} hCG was revealed to encourage sperm penetration into perivitelline space even in oocytes without cumulus cells. 10 IU ml^{-1} hCG and 2 μg ml^{-1} progesterone was also suggested to encourage fertilization (sperm–egg fusion) both in cumulus-enclosed and cumulus-free oocytes. It can be stated that hCG and progesterone may have some direct effect on zona pellucida or vitellus.

Part II

Section 3
Ovulation and Fertilization

16
Electron microscopic observations on ovarian perifollicular vessels in indomethacin-treated rabbits

H. KANZAKI, Y. OKUDA, K. TAKEMORI, N. KAWAMURA and H. OKAMURA

The relationship between the prostaglandins (PGs) and ovulation has been suggested by many investigators. It is well known that ovulation in the rabbit can be blocked by administration of indomethacin (IM)[1], an inhibitor of PG biosynthesis[2]. In order to clarify the vascular changes at ovulation–inhibition by IM, we observed perifollicular vessels of the rabbit ovary after treatment with hCG and IM by casting/SEM[3] and TEM combined with carbon tracers[4].

MATERIALS AND METHODS

Twenty mature Japanese white female rabbits were examined sequentially after the treatment with hCG (100 IU) and IM (20 mg kg^{-1}). The ovaries were perfused and vascular casts were made, using Mercox resin for SEM observation. In a group of the rabbits, carbon particles (Günther Wagner, Pelikan Werke, Hannover, Germany, batch no. cl1/1431a, 0.15 ml kg^{-1}, 20–30 nm diameter) were injected via the aorta at each time interval after hCG/IM as a tracer for the investigation of capillary permeability, and the walls of prominent follicles were excised and embedded for TEM observation. These SEM and TEM observations were compared with those of the normal ovulatory process[3,4].

RESULTS

SEM observations; 4 and 6 hours after the hCG/IM treatment, some of the Graafian follicles were enlarged, but the three-dimensional vascular pattern surrounding the follicles was similar to those of the normal ovulatory process. At 12 hours, some of the follicles were enlarged up to 1.5 mm in diameter, and the upper part of the follicles was protruded beyond the surface of the ovary (Figure 1). However, resin leakage from the thecal capillary plexus and incomplete castings of the apical vessels, which are characteristic findings in the wall of control pre-ruptured follicles (Figure 2)[3], were not observed. TEM observations; in IM-treated rabbit ovaries, carbon tracers were confined to the thecal capillary lumen all through this experiment. The interendothelial gaps of the capillary, which had been constantly observed in the normal ovulatory process[4], were never found out after 12 hours (Figure 3). On the contrary, the carbon tracers had been leaking through the interendothelial gaps in the walls of pre-ruptured large follicles 10 hours after hCG treatment alone (Figure 4).

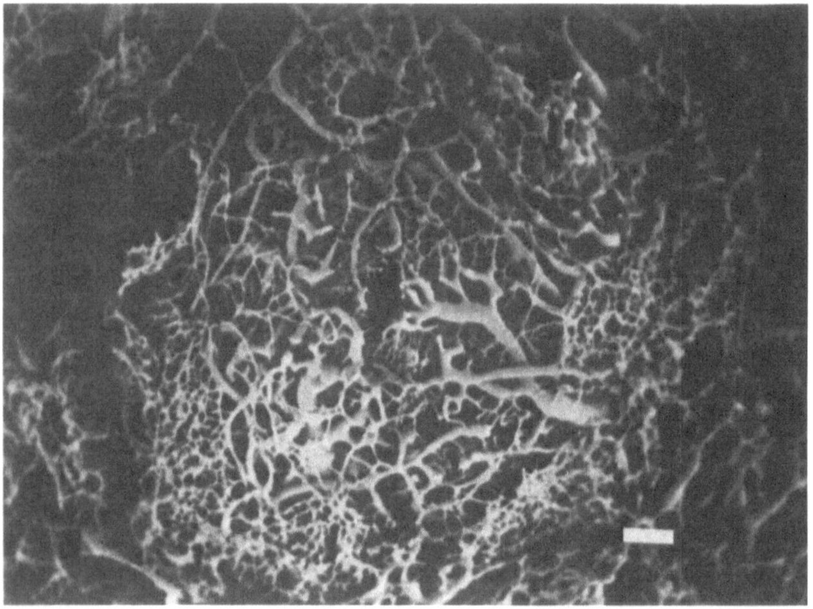

Figure 1 SEM of a vascular cast of a follicle 12 hours after hCG/IM treatment. Bar = 100 μm

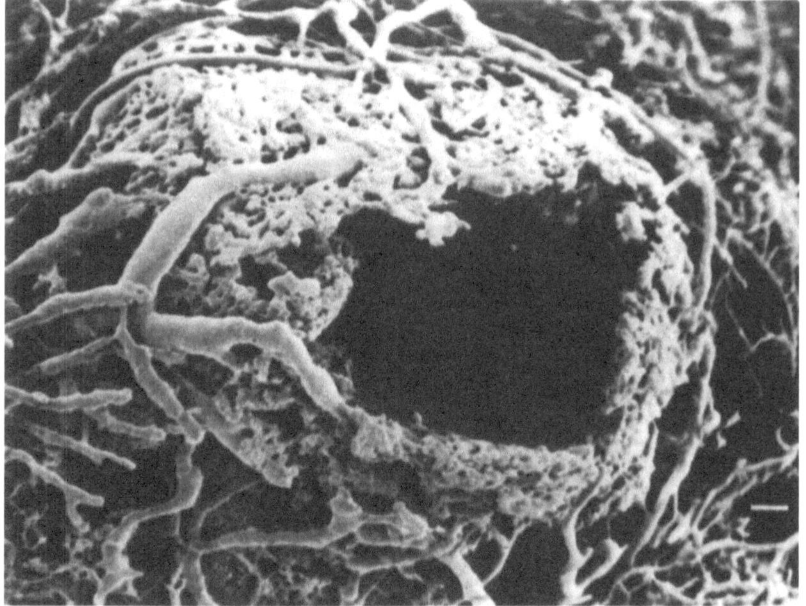

Figure 2 SEM of a follicular cast 10 hours after hCG treatment. Bar = 100 μm

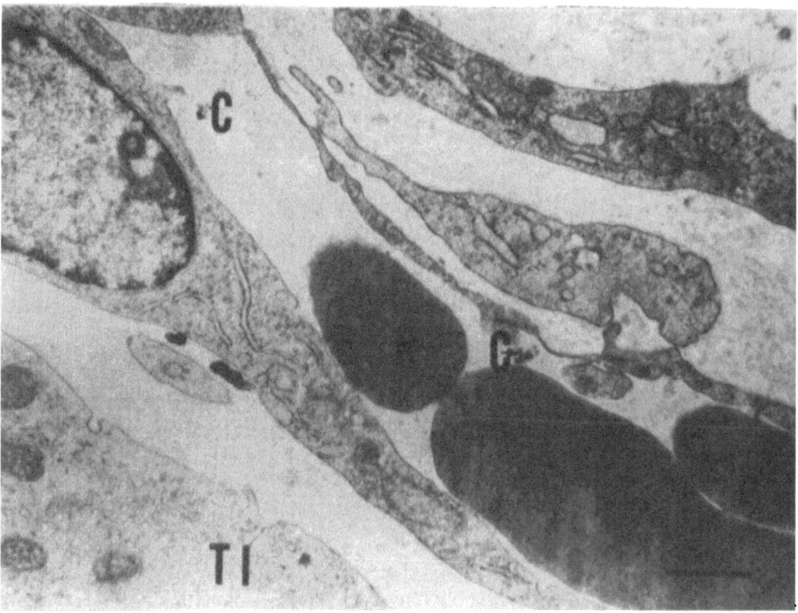

Figure 3 TEM of a thecal capillary wall 12 hours after hCG/IM treatment. Bar = 1 μm. C = Carbon particles; R = red blood cells; TI = theca interna cell

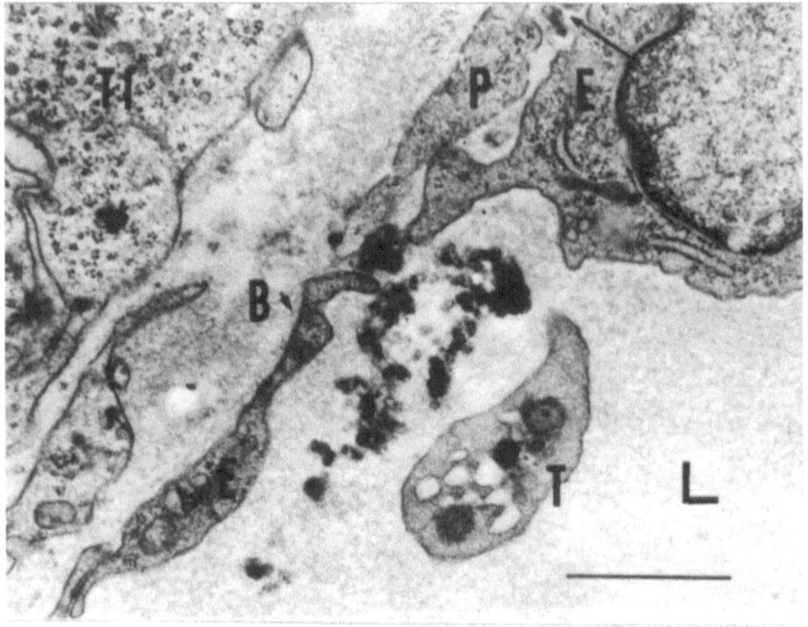

Figure 4 TEM of a thecal capillary wall 10 hours after hCG treatment. Bar = 1 μm. L = Capillary lumen; E = endothelial cell; P = pericyte; B = capillary basement membrane; TI = theca interna cell

DISCUSSION

Casting/SEM observations revealed that the vascular pattern surrounding the follicles was essentially unchanged, and no resin leakage was observed even after 12 hours in the ovaries of hCG/IM treated rabbits. The capillary fenestrations and formation of interendothelial gaps, which were observed in the normal ovulatory process, were never seen in the thecal capillaries. These findings indicate that the increase of capillary permeability, which occurs prior to follicle rupture in the thecal capillaries, is dependent on PGs and is mandatory in the normal mechanism of follicle rupture.

References

1. O'Grady, J.P., Caldwall, B.V., Auletta, F.J. and Speroff, L. (1972). The effects of an inhibitor of prostaglandin synthesis (indomethacin) on ovulation, pregnancy and pseudopregnancy in the rabbit. *Prostaglandins*, **1**, 97
2. Vane, J.R. (1971). Inhibition of prostaglandin synthesis as a mechanism of action for aspirin-like drugs. *Nature (New Biol.)*, **231**, 232

3. Kanzaki, H., Okamura, H., Okuda, Y., Takenaka, A., Morimoto, K. and Nishimura, T. (1982). Scanning electron microscopic study of rabbit ovarian follicle microvasculature using resin injection-corrosion casts. *J. Anat.*, **134**, 697
4. Okuda, Y., Okamura, H., Kanzaki, H., Takenaka, A., Morimoto, K. and Nishimura, T. (1980). An ultrastructural study of capillary permeability of perifollicular capillaries of rabbit ovary during ovulation using carbon particles as a tracer. *Acta Obstet. Gynecol. Jpn.*, **32**, 859

17
Monoclonal antibodies to porcine zona pellucida antigens and their inhibitory effects on fertilization

S. ISOJIMA, K. KOYAMA, A. HASEGAWA, Y. TSUNODA and A. HANADA

In order to study the blocking effect of monoclonal antibody (Moab) to porcine zona pellucida (ZP) on fertilization in pig and other mammals, the production of hybridomas to porcine ZP was attempted.

Male BALB/c mice were immunized with an emulsion obtained from ZP and complete Freund's adjuvant and the spleen cells (7.8×10^7) of immunized mice were fused with mouse myeloma cells (7.8×10^6, P3U1) in the presence of polyethylene glycol as described in our previous report[1]. After HAT selection, the supernatant of the medium in each well containing growing hybrid cells was examined for antibody activity to porcine ZP by immunofluorescent staining. After limiting dilution method of antibody positive cell lines, five hybridoma cell lines were established by cloning. The immunoglobulin classes were IgG2a from hybridoma B11C8 and IgM from the other four.

By indirect immunofluorescent staining, all five Moabs stained only oocytes and no other organ tissues from pigs. When slices of porcine ovary were stained with FITC, only the ZP was clearly stained and no other regions of the ovary such as stroma cells, theca cells and follicular cells could be stained. These results suggest that the Moabs were tissue specific to zona antigens of porcine oocytes.

Cross-distribution of the zona antigen among species such as pig, human, hamster, rat and mouse was examined by FITC staining with these five Moabs to porcine ZP. Moabs from hybridoma C6H1, D3H4 and G10F9 all clearly stained ZP or vitelline membrane from humans, hamsters, rats and mice; but that from hybridoma G10G5 stained only ZP from hamsters besides pigs. Moab from B11C8 was species specific and only stained porcine ZP. These results demonstrate that the porcine ZP contained a number of cross-reactive antigens among species and the distribution of particular antigens was quite different in each species. The localization of a certain common antigen to porcine ZP in oocyte was not uniform among these species. The γ-globulin of the conventional rabbit anti-porcine ZP antiserum stained ZPe of pigs, humans, hamsters, rats and mice evenly, but the Moab of B11C8 stained only porcine ZP. The Moab of G10G5 could stain ZPe of pigs and hamsters; but ZPe of humans, rats and mice were not stained by this Moab. It is interesting that the Moab of G10F9 stained ZPe of pigs and humans and also stained vitelline membranes of hamsters, rats and mice. The Moab of C6H1 stained only the vitelline membrane of oocytes in all species except humans, whose ZP was evenly stained weakly, though the inner layer of ZP was strongly stained. The staining of oocytes in hamsters and rats by Moabs of G6H1 and D3H4 was rather granular.

When porcine oocytes were treated with conventional antiserum to porcine ZP, the binding of boar spermatozoa on the zona surface was completely blocked. However, the inhibitory effect of each Moab on sperm-binding to the zona surface varied. As shown in Table 1, the Moab from hybridoma B11C8 which was species specific to pig showed the strongest inhibitory effect on sperm binding among the five Moabs examined. The Moab from G10F9 which stained porcine and human ZPe but only the vitelline membrane of hamsters, rats and mice by FITC, indicated the second strongest inhibitory effect on sperm binding. Moab from G10G5, however, did not demonstrate any effect on sperm binding.

Table 2 shows the effect of Moabs on *in vitro* fertilization (IVF) of hamster oocytes. The conventional anti-porcine ZP antiserum completely blocked IVF of hamster oocytes, but none of the five Moabs to porcine ZP showed any inhibitory effect on IVF of hamster oocytes. When Moabs from both G10G5 and G10F9 were applied for the treatment of hamster oocytes, no inhibitory effects on IVF were observed. However, when the treatment of hamster oocytes with Moab from G10G5 was followed by anti-mouse γ-globulin serum, the distinct inhibition of IVF was observed as shown in Table 3. In this case, a light-scattering precipitin ring on the surface of ZP was observed.

Table 1 Effect of monoclonal antibodies to zona pellucida on binding of boar spermatozoa to pig oocytes

Antibody	*No. of examined eggs*	*No. (±SD) of bound sperm/egg*	*Range*
None	79	16.0 ± 14.0	1–65
C2D8	41	20.0 ± 14.1	1–72
Conventional	29	0	0
B11C8	27	1.3 ± 1.1	0–6☆
C6H1	44	7.5 ± 6.7	0–25☆
D3H4	50	8.7 ± 7.5	0–31☆☆
G10G5	31	45.5 ± 38.5	3–150
G10F9	28	2.1 ± 1.5	0–8☆

Significantly different from control (None): ★ $p<0.01$; ★★ $p<0.05$.

Table 2 Effect of monoclonal antibodies to zona pellucida on *in vitro* fertilization of hamster oocytes

Antibody	*No. of examined eggs*	*No. (%) of fertilized eggs*
B11C8	27	25 (93)
Conventional	14	0
C6H1	22	17 (77)
D3H4	22	19 (86)
G10G5	44	36 (82)
G10F9	28	27 (94)
G10G5 + G10F9	17	13 (76)

Table 3 Effect of simultaneous use of monoclonal antibodies to zona pellucida and anti-mouse immunoglobulin antibody on *in vitro* fertilization of hamster oocytes

Antibody	*No. of examined eggs*	*No. (%) of fertilized eggs*
P3U1	20	20 (100)
C6H1	25	22 (88)
D3H4	27	23 (85)
G10G5	30	9 (30*)
G10F9	26	26 (100)

* Significantly different from control (P3U1)

Reference

1. Isojima, S., Koyama, K. and Hasegawa, A. (1981). Production of monoclonal antibody to zona pellucida from porcine oocytes. *Acta Obstet. Gynecol. Jpn.*, **33**, 1995

18
Histochemistry of hydroxysteroid dehydrogenase activities of *in vitro* fertilized eggs of rabbit

K. MIYAZAKI and O. SUGIMOTO

In order to investigate the steroidogenesis of fertilized eggs, hydroxysteroid dehydrogenase (Δ^5-3β-HSD,17β-HSD) activities were examined histochemically in rabbit eggs, which were fertilized *in vivo* or *in vitro* and subsequently cultured *in vivo* or *in vitro*, respectively.

There was no difference in HSD activities among these eggs in each combination until 4 days after fertilization. However, on day 6, Δ^5-3β-HSD activity with pregnenolone (Δ^5-p) as a substrate and 17β-HSD activity with oestradiol-17β (E_2) as a substrate tended to reduce.

Results of the present experiments (Tables 1–3) suggested that HSD activities in rabbit eggs were autonomous at least from fertilization to the initial genetic stage; and that steroidogenesis, such as production of progestin and oestrogen, was reduced on day 6 in eggs fertilized and cultured *in vitro*. Since the same results were obtained in eggs fertilized *in vivo* and cultured *in vitro* on day 6, the reduction of these enzyme activities did not seem directly associated with *in vitro* fertilization but rather with influence of the long-term culture that differed from the maternal environment.

Table 1 Hydroxysteroid dehydrogenase activities in rabbit eggs fertilized *in vivo*

Enzyme	*Substrate*	*Day 1 (24 h pc)*	*Day 2 (48 h pc)*	*Day 4 (96 h pc)*	*Day 6 (144 h pc)*
3β-HSD	DHA	++	+	++	++
	Δ^5-P	−	−	+	++
17β-HSD	E_2	−	−	+	++
	T	+	+	++	++

pc = Post coitally.
DHA = Dehydroepiandrosterone; T = testosterone.

Table 2 Hydroxysteroid dehydrogenase activities in rabbit eggs fertilized *in vitro**

Enzyme	*Substrate*	*Day 1 (12 h)*	*Day 2 (36 h)*	*Day 4 (84 h)*	*Day 6 (132 h)*
3β-HSD	DHA	++	+	++	++
	Δ^5-P	−	−	+	+
17β-HSD	E_2	−	−	+	+
	T	+	+	++	++

* Times refer to period after fertilization.
DHA = Dehydroepiandrosterone; T = testosterone.

Table 3 Hydroxysteroid dehydrogenase activities in rabbit eggs at day 6

Enzyme	*Substrate*	*In vivo fertilization in vivo culture*	*In vitro fertilization*	*In vitro culture and in vivo fertilization*
3β-HSD	DHA	++	++	++
	Δ^5-P	++	+	+
17β-HSD	E_2	++	+	+
	T	++	++	++

DHA = Dehydroepiandrosterone: T = testosterone.

Part III

Semen and Spermatozoa

Part III

Section 1
Animal Studies

19
Analysis of the outer acrosomal membrane of boar spermatozoa by biochemical and immunological methods

E. TÖPFER-PETERSEN, F. KRASSNIGG and W.-B. SCHILL

For mammalian spermatozoa the fertilization process is associated with a variety of structural and biochemical changes occurring during epididymal transit and after ejaculation during its residence in the female reproductive tract. During the last decade the molecular changes of the plasma membrane accompanying sperm maturation[1] and capacitation[2] were investigated for several species leading to valuable information on mammalian fertilization. By two-dimensional electrophoresis combined with sensitive staining procedures more than 250 proteins and glycoproteins could be discriminated[3,4] indicating the complexity of the sperm membranes which correlates with the heterogeneous functional capabilities of the spermatozoon.

However, little is known about structure and function of the acrosomal membranes and their changes correlated with capacitation and acrosome reaction. The possibility of isolating the outer acrosomal membrane (OAM) from boar spermatozoa tempted us, first to start with the investigations of this membrane in order to characterize the mammalian acrosome.

Homogenization and gradient centrifugation through colloidal silica rendered a largely homogeneous membrane fraction which contains lipids and proteins in equimolar amounts and 5–10% carbohydrates. By means of gas chromatography all carbohydrates commonly found in glycoproteins such as mannose, galactose, *N*-acetylglucosamine, *N*-acetylgalactosamine, sialic acid and small amounts of fucose could be determined[5,6]. The carbohydrate content of the plasma membrane and the inner acrosomal membrane was demonstrated by their lectin interaction for several species[7]. However, the carbohydrate content seems most controversial and consequently so does the lectin-binding ability of the outer acrosomal membrane. By electron-microscopical examinations of boar spermatozoa using the lectin-peroxidase and lectin-ferritin technique it could be demonstrated that the OAM contains binding sites for concanavalin A (Con A) and Ricinus communis-agglutinin-120 (RCA-120)[8]. RCA-120 binds preferentially to the exposed terminal galactose of carbohydrate side-chains. These galactose residues could be easily radiolabelled with tritium thus facilitating the detection of RCA receptor proteins. In the case of the OAM, tritium was incorporated by the galactose oxidase-3-H-borohydride procedure exclusively into a 340 kdalton protein, which even after reduction has a molecular weight of about 270 kdalton. Moreover, this major OAM galactoprotein could be shown to possess binding sites for Con A.

Screening for mannose-containing proteins was achieved by means of an enzyme-linked-lectin-assay (ELLA) specifically developed for the sensitive detection of Con A (and other lectins) binding properties throughout chromatography and electrophoresis. By affinity chromatography, HPLC and SDS-PAGE, four further Con A receptor proteins corresponding to molecular weights of about 120, 110, 88 and 66 kdaltons could be identified and partially isolated. Conspicuously, most of the low molecular weight proteins (20 kdaltons) contain no carbohydrates[9].

For immunological localization and physiological studies an antiserum against the isolated OAM was raised in rabbits and the IgG fraction was isolated by immunoabsorption chromatography. The isolated antibodies observed by indirect immunofluorescence bind exclusively to the acrosomal cap of the boar sperm head indicating the acrosomal origin of the membrane fraction[10]. A distinct antibody precipitation at the OAM visualized for transmission electron microscopy using the immunoferritin technique demonstrated that in fact predominantly antigenic structures of the OAM will be recognized by the rabbit antibodies[11].

Immunoprecipitation of the ^{3}H- and ^{125}I-labelled OAM followed by analysis on SDS-PAGE gave preliminary information about the components being recognized by the anti-OAM-IgG. Beside the [^{3}H]galactoprotein (340 kdalton) only some low molecular weight ^{125}I-proteins (20 kdalton) could be identified showing the limits of this radiolabelling procedure[10]. By high-resolution gel filtration and electro-phoresis combined with the ELISA technique immunoreaction with all major OAM-proteins could be demonstrated (unpublished obser-vations).

Of course, the overall question is: what are the functions of distinct OAM-proteins and glycoproteins. The isolation and purification of single membrane proteins for the production of antibodies needed for functional studies is a very time- and material-consuming work. Therefore, the production of monoclonal antibodies was initiated according to the hybridoma technique[12].

After 5–6 months' immunization of Balb/C mice a strong positive antiserum was obtained, which reacted exclusively with the acrosomal cap of the boar sperm head and showed an extremely good cross-reaction with human spermatozoa when assayed by indirect immunofluorescence. One fusion resulted in about 100 ELISA positive cultures of which about 28 reacted positively with human spermatozoa. So far, 20 hybridoma culture supernatants were tested by indirect immunofluorescence and a combined HPLC-ELISA-system leading to the following results.

Three hybridoma cultures (L81, L264, L234) were observed to generate a distinct 'patchwork-like' fluorescence at the anterior part of the head indicating perhaps the distribution of antigenic sites in discrete domains of the OAM. One of them (L234) showed a cross-reaction with human spermatozoa. High-resolution gel filtration of the solubilized OAM on three TSK-HPLC columns connected in series separated the OAM polypeptides according to their molecular weights. Testing the eluates by ELISA, the anti-mouse-serum showed immunoreaction over the whole separation range of the columns due to the complexity of antigenic structures, whereas each of the four hybridoma culture supernatants generated a typical ELISA pattern giving first information on the corresponding antigens. With L268, which showed no significant immunofluorescence, antigenic structures were detected by HPLC-ELISA analysis in the high molecular weight region. This might be due to the fact that antigenic structures of the high molecular weight proteins are protected within the membrane unit.

Under the light of these preliminary results we now concentrate our effort on analysing predominantly the cross-reacting hybridoma cultures, which enables us to introduce porcine OAM-antibodies into human fertilization studies.

Acknowledgement

This work was supported by Deutsche Forschungsgemeinschaft Schi 86/7–4.

References

1. Nicolson, G.L. and Yanagimachi, R. (1979). Cell surface changes associated with epididymal maturation of mammalian spermatozoa. In Fawcett, D.W. and Bedford, J.M. (eds.) *The Spermatozoon.* p. 187. (Baltimore: Urban and Schwarzenberg)
2. O'Rand, M.G. (1979). Changes in the sperm surface properties correlated with capacitation. In Fawcett, D.W. and Bedford, J.M. (eds.) *The Spermatozoon.* p. 195. (Baltimore: Urban and Schwarzenberg)
3. Peterson, R.N., Russell, L.D., Hunt, W., Bundman, D. and Freund, M. (1983). Characterization of boar sperm plasma membranes by two-dimensional PAGE and isolation of specific groups of polypeptides by anion exchange chromatography and lectin affinity chromatography. *J. Androl.*, **4**, 71
4. Russell, L.D., Peterson, R.N., Russell, T.A. and Hunt, W. (1983). Electrophoretic map of boar sperm plasma membrane polypeptides and localization and fractionation of specific polypeptide subclasses. *Biol. Reprod.*, **28**, 393
5. Töpfer-Petersen, E. and Schill, W.-B. (1981). A new separation method of subcellular fractions of boar spermatozoa. *Andrologia*, **13**, 174
6. Töpfer-Petersen,E., Schmoeckel, C. and Schill, W.-B. (1983). The acrosomal membrane system of boar spermatozoa – morphological and biochemical studies. *Andrologia*, **15**, 197
7. Koehler, J. (1981). Lectins as probes of the spermatozoon surface. *Arch. Androl.*, **6**, 197
8. Töpfer-Petersen, E., Januschke, E., Schmoeckel, C. and Schill, W.-B. (1984). Ultrastructural localization of lectin binding sites in the acrosomal membrane system of boar spermatozoa. *Andrologia* (In press)
9. Töpfer-Petersen, E. and Schill, W.-B. (1984). Characterization of lectin receptors isolated from the outer acrosomal membrane of boar spermatozoa. *Int. J. Androl.* **6**, 375
10. Hinrichsen-Kohane, A.C., Töpfer-Petersen, E., Dietl, T. and Schill, W.-B. (1984). Immunological characterization of the outer acrosomal membrane of boar spermatozoa. *Gamete Res.* (In press)
11. Töpfer-Petersen, E., Hinrichsen-Kohane, A.C., Schmoeckel, C. and Schill, W.-B. (1984). The acrosomal membrane system and its role in mammalian fertilization. In Völter (ed.) *Proceedings of the 4th German–Russian Symposium on The Chemistry of Peptides and Proteins. Vol. 2.* (Berlin: Walter de Gruyter)(In press)
12. Koehler, G. and Milstein, C. (1975). Continuous cultures of fused cells secreting antibodies of predefined specificity. *Nature (Lond.)*, **256**, 495

20
A new acrosin inhibitor in boar seminal plasma

D. ČECHOVÁ, L. VESELSKÝ and V. JONÁKOVÁ

Protease inhibitors are proteins capable of inhibiting the activity of proteolytic enzymes in the organism. Proteases participate in important biological processes (protein synthesis, proteolysis, fibrinolysis, inflammatory processes, immunological defence and fertilization). By limiting protease activities, protease inhibitors can help to regulate these processes. Many authors have demonstrated the presence of protease inhibitors in seminal plasma, in acid extract of ejaculated spermatozoa and on the surface of sperm cell membranes[1,2]. In the male genital tract, protease inhibitors are secreted by the tissues of the seminal vesicles, the vas deferens, the epididymis, the urethra, the ampullae and the testes[3,4]. The physiological significance of protease inhibitors is that they protect the tissues and sperm cells from proteolytic degradation by proteinases released after destruction of the cell membranes of dead spermatozoa[1]. They may further have the role of protecting the tissues from the action of granulocytic proteases released during inflammatory processes[5]. It was demonstrated that proteins antigenically identical with inhibitors isolated from colostrum and seminal plasma are present on the surface of leukocytes[6].

The aim of the present study was to isolate from boar seminal plasma a new protease inhibitor immunologically similar to the protease inhibitor isolated from the organs of cattle (Trasylol). It was also hoped, using immunological methods, to determine its distribution in the tissues of the genital tract and on the spermatozoa.

Antibodies against the Trasylol–trypsin inhibitor isolated from bovine lung tissue (TKI) were prepared by immunizing rabbits. Immunoelectrophoresis and radial immunodiffusion showed that boar seminal plasma reacted with these antibodies. The immunoglobulin fraction was isolated from TKI antiserum by the batch method on DEAE cellulose suspended in 0.01 mol l^{-1} phosphate buffer at pH 7.5 containing 0.015 mol l^{-1} NaC1. The separated immunoglobulin fraction was lyophilized and was absorbed to CNBr-activated Sepharose 4 B in a concentration of 10 mg protein to 1 ml Sepharose. The immunosorbent with absorbed anti-TKI antibodies allowed the isolation, from boar seminal plasma and seminal vesicle fluid, of a protein inhibiting the enzymatic activity of trypsin, acrosin, plasmin and chymotrypsin, but not kallikrein (Figure 1). The molecular weight was estimated as 13 000 by gel filtration on a column (0.5 × 110 cm) of Sephadex G-50 equilibrated with 0.1 mol l^{-1} sodium acetate pH 4 (Figure 2).

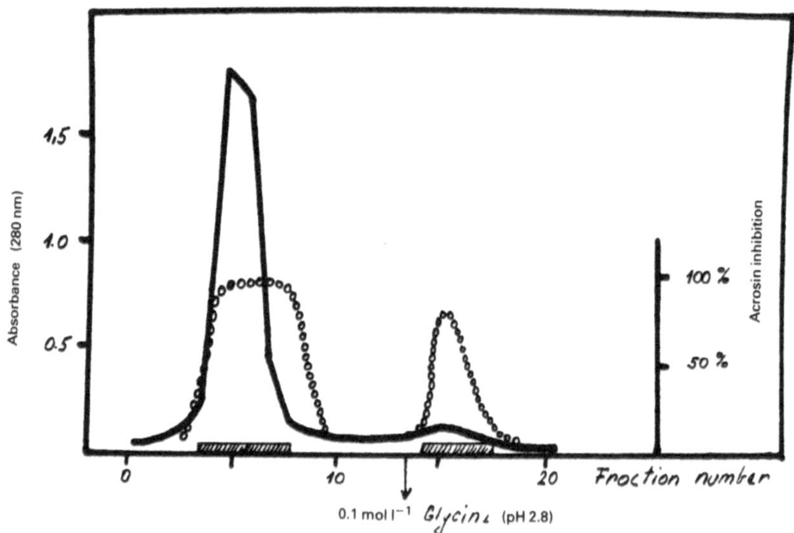

Figure 1 Isolation of seminal vesicle inhibitor on the CNBr activated Sepharose 4 B (2 × 10 cm) with adsorbed anti-TKI antibodies. Elution was performed at a flow rate of 40 ml h^{-1} with 0.1 mol l^{-1} glycine pH 2.8. ooooooo = Acrosin inhibition; ——— = absorbance (280 nm)

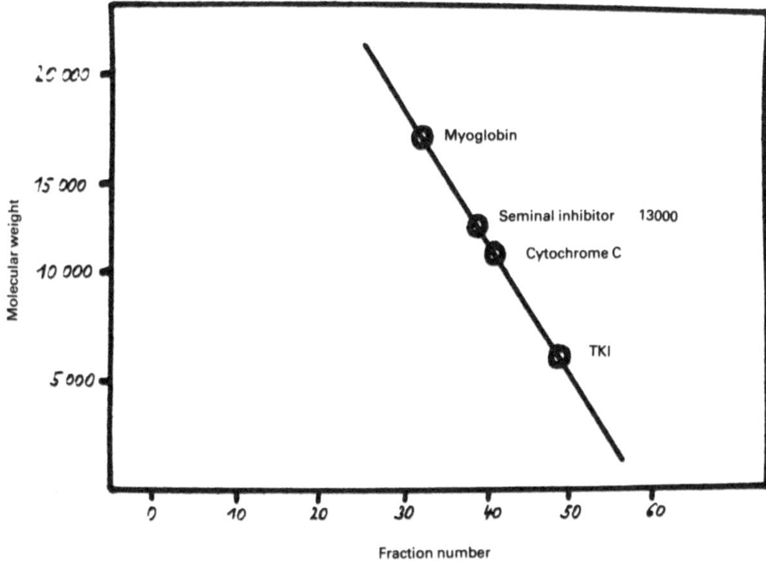

Figure 2 The molecular weight was estimated on a column of Sephadex G-50 (0.5 × 110 cm) equilibrated with 0.1 mol l^{-1} sodium acetate pH 4 at a flow rate of 5 ml h^{-1}

Immunoelectrophoresis and radial immunodiffusion detected one precipitation zone in the reaction of TKI antiserum with 1% TKI solution; the same zone was found in the reaction of this antiserum with boar seminal plasma and boar seminal vesicle fluid (Figure 3). The reaction with bull, rabbit and ram seminal plasma and with 2–5% solutions of the lyophilized fluids of bull seminal vesicles, ampullae and cauda epididymis was negative. This antiserum likewise reacted negatively with 2–5% solutions of the lyophilized fluids of boar prostate, cauda epididymis and rete testis. In absorption tests, anti-TKI antibodies were absorbed only by boar seminal plasma, seminal vesicle fluid or thrice-washed ejaculated spermatozoa.

An indirect immunofluorescence test confirmed the immunoprecipitation results. After administering TKI antiserum, immunofluorescence was found only on tissue sections of boar seminal vesicles (Figure 4). Anti-TKI antibodies also reacted with antigens on ejaculated boar spermatozoa. No fluorescence of boar epididymal sperm cells or bull spermatozoa was observed.Fluorescence of boar seminal vesicle tissue sections and ejaculated spermatozoa was inhibited only if TKI antiserum

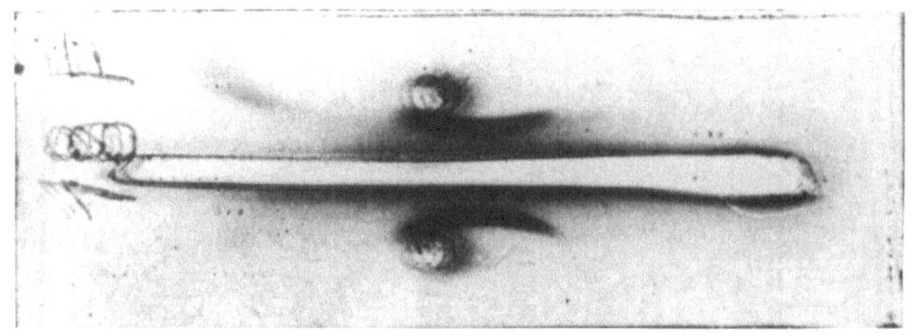

Figure 3 Above: the immunoelectrophoretic reaction of antisera to TKI with homologous antigen. Below: the reaction of antisera to TKI with seminal vesicle fluid

was absorbed by boar seminal vesicle fluid, ejaculated sper-matozoa and lyophilized TKI (20 mg to 1 ml antiserum). The survey of cross-reactions of antisera to TKI with various genital tract fluids and cells is given in Table 1.

Table 1 Results of cross-reactions of TKI antisera with various genital tract fluids and cells

Animal	*Antigen*	*Immuno-precipitation (fluids)*	*Immuno-fluorescence (tissues)*
Boar	Seminal plasma	+	
	Seminal vesicle	+	+
	Prostate	–	–
	Epididymis	–	–
	Rete testis	–	
	Urethra		–
	Ejaculated spermatozoa		+
	Epididymal spermatozoa		–
	Rete testis spermatozoa		–
	Blood plasma	–	
Bull	Seminal plasma	–	
	Spermatozoa		–
	Blood plasma	–	
Ram	Seminal plasma	–	
Rabbit	Seminal plasma	–	
	TKI 1 %	+	

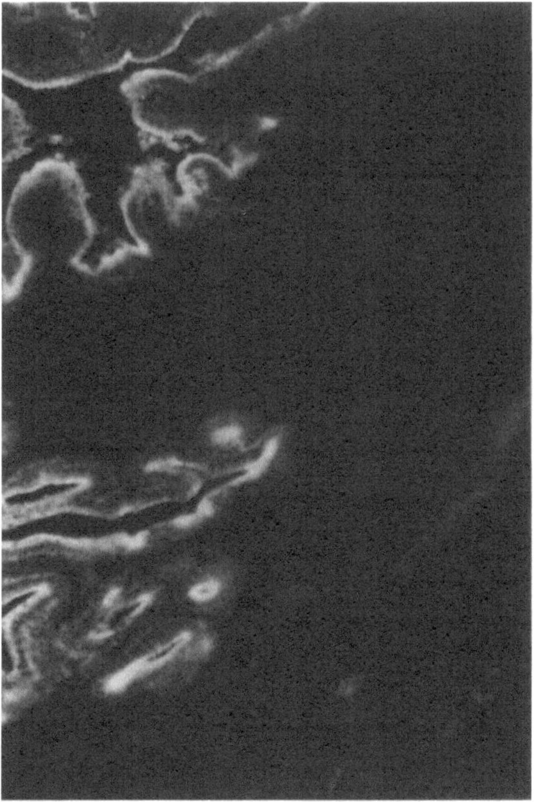

Figure 4 Immunofluorescence of antisera to TKI with the tissue section of boar seminal vesicles. × 240

The inhibitor investigated in the present study probably belongs to the group of inhibitors structurally homologous with Kunitz's basic inhibitor from the pancreas. It is the first inhibitor of this type to be described as specific for the reproductive tract. Our laboratory will continue to study its properties.

References

1. Fritz, H., Schiessler, H., Schill, W.B., Tschesche, H., Heimburger, N. and Wallner, O. (1975). Low molecular weight proteinase (Acrosin) inhibitors from human and boar seminal plasma and spermatozoa and human cervical mucus – isolation, properties and biological aspects. In Reich, E., Rifkin, D.B. and Shaw, E. (eds.) *Proteases and Biological Control.* pp. 737–66. (New York: Cold Spring Harbor)
2. Hartree, E.F. (1977). Spermatozoa, eggs and proteinases. *Biochem. Soc. Trans.*, **5**, 375

3. Suominen, J. and Setchell, B.P. (1972). Enzymes and trypsin inhibitors in the rete testis fluid of rams and boars. *J. Reprod. Fertil.*, **30**, 235
4. Veselský, L. and Čechová, D. (1980). Distribution of acrosin inhibitors in bull reproductive tissues and spermatozoa. *Hoppe-Seyler's Z. Physiol. Chem.*, **361**, 715
5. Fritz, H. (1980). Proteinase inhibitors in severe inflammatory processes/septic shock and experimental endotoxemia/biochemical, pathophysical and therapeutic aspects. In *Protein Degradation in Health and Diseases.* Ciba Foundation 75. pp. 351–79. (Amsterdam: Excerpta Medica ISBN Elsevier North Holland)
6. Veselský, L., Čechová, D., Hruban, V. and Klaudy, J. (1982). Seminal and colostral protease inhibitors on leucocytes. *Hoppe Seyler's Z. Physiol. Chem.*, **363**, 113

Part III

Section 2
Practical Aspects of Human Semen Quality

21
A 'migration–gravity sedimentation' method for collecting motile spermatozoa from human semen

N.T. TEA, M. JONDET and R. SCHOLLER

Methods of separating motile human spermatozoa avoiding centrifugation have been described[1–3]. Ejaculated semen is deposited in contact with the culture medium, and then motile spermatozoa migrate upward into the supernatant, where they must be collected within 1 or 2 hours before their sedimentation. A simple new method which combines both the migration and the sedimentation phenomena has been developed[4].

MATERIALS AND METHODS

The apparatus using the migration–sedimentation (MS) technique is shown in Figure 1. It is made of two built-in concentric tubes in which the progressive spermatozoa 'jump over' the edge of the central tube. Then they sediment at the bottom of the central conical tube where they can be collected by aspiration.

The semen specimens were obtained by masturbation from normo- and oligo-asthenozoospermic patients, and from husbands involved in the *in vitro* fertilization (IVF) programme. The IVF procedure has been described elsewhere[5]. Semen analysis[6] was performed on aliquots removed before and after the MS procedure.

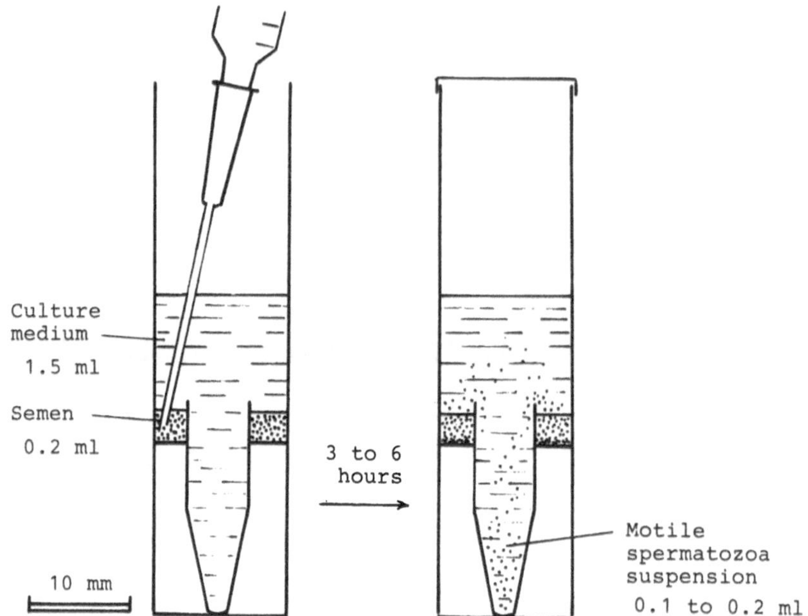

Figure 1 Apparatus (patented) for collecting motile spermatozoa. The prototype model has been made of Pyrex glass. The tubes are filled with B2 medium (API System, France). A sterile 1 ml syringe is used to deposit semen sample at the bottom of the medium in the outer tube. The semen/medium interface must be at 1 mm beneath the edge of the inner tube. Incubation is carried out at 37°C during 30 min, and then completed at room temperature (≈ 20°C) during 3–6 h. Sperm suspension can be collected by aspiration from the conical tube

RESULTS AND DISCUSSION

As shown in Figure 2, in both normozoospermic and asthenozoospermic specimens the percentage of motility increased to 98% and was maintained at that level for at least 3–6 hours after the MS procedure. The motility then did not decrease until 24 hours later. On the other hand, in the control ejaculated semen, there was a rapid decrease of motility during the same time period. This would demonstrate that collected spermatozoa in the medium are protected against the deleterious effects of seminal plasma[7].

Thirteen ejaculates have been tested. The average number (with ranges in parentheses) of motile spermatozoa in the 0.2 ml ejaculate was $8.3 \times 10^6 (2.2–13.0 \times 10^6)$ and in the 0.2 ml collected sperm suspension

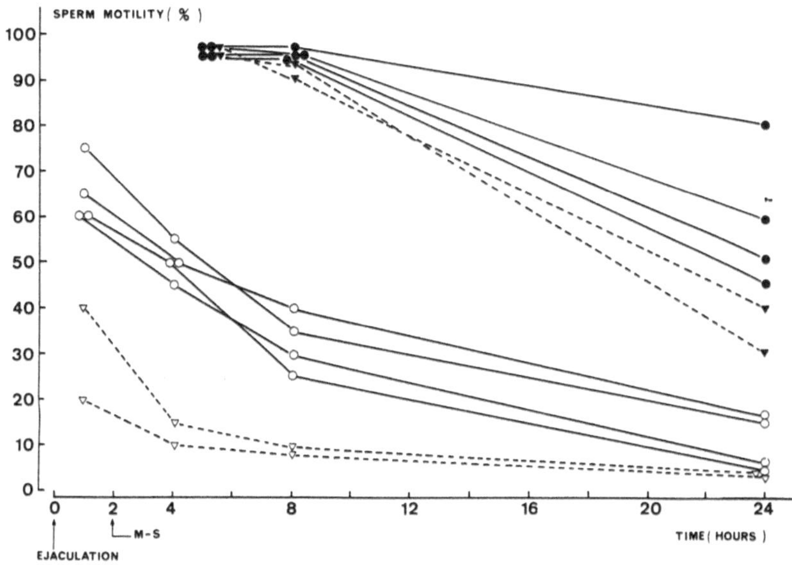

Figure 2 Comparison of percentages of sperm motility in the control ejaculated semen from four normo- (o — o) and two asthenozoospermic (△—△) subjects with those observed in the medium collected by the MS method (●—●, ▲—▲)

was 5.1 × 10^6(1.3–12.3 × 10^6). This represented a mean recovery rate of 58%. There was an average of 51% (35–70%) motile spermatozoa in the ejaculate, and 93% (85–98%) in the collected sperm suspension after the MS procedure. Abnormal forms decreased from 36% in the ejaculate to 21% in the MS tube.

Spermatozoa collected by this MS method have good viability and are freed of other cellular particles and debris.

Preliminary results in IVF show that 11 oocytes, out of 18 collected from eight patients, were fertilized and divided into embryos of two or more cells. It is important to note that at least one oocyte per patient has been fertilized, in spite of three husbands with asthenozoospermia and one with oligo-asthenozoospermia.

Intrauterine artificial insemination with MS collected spermatozoa from fresh ejaculates or from freezing semen are presently being investigated in our laboratory.

References

1. Lopata, A., Patullo, M.J., Chang, A. and James, B. (1976). A method for collecting motile spermatozoa from human semen. *Fertil. Steril.*, **27**, 677

2. Harris, S.J., Milligan, M.P., Masson, G.M. and Dennis, K.J. (1981). Improved separation of motile sperm in asthenospermia and its application to artificial insemination homologous. *Fertil. Steril.*, **36**, 219
3. Mortimer, D., Leslie, E.E., Kelly, R.W. and Templeton, A.A. (1982). Morphological selection of human spermatozoa *in vivo* and *in vitro*. *J. Reprod. Fertil.*, **64**, 391
4. Tea, N.T., Jondet, M. and Scholler, R. (1983). Procédé d'isolement de spermatozoides mobiles du sperme humain par la méthode de migration-sédimentation. *Path. Biol.* **31**, 688
5. Dominique, S., Cornier, E., Jondet, M. and Scholler, R. (1983). Fécondation *in vitro* et replacement: résultats préliminaires. *Path. Biol.* **31**, 693
6. Jondet, M. and Tea, N.T. (1980). Le spermogramme et son interprétation. In Scholler, R. (ed.) *Hormonologie de la Stérilité*. pp. 223–52. (Paris: SEPE)
7. Eliasson, R., Johnsen, O. and Lindholmer, C. (1974). Effects of seminal plasma on some functional properties of human spermatozoa. In Mancini, R.E. and Martini, L. (eds.) *Male Fertility and Sterility*. pp. 107–21. (London: Academic Press)

22
The influence of semen quality on *in vitro* fertilization of human oocytes

K. DIEDRICH, H. VAN DER VEN, S. AL-HASANI, U. HAMERICH, F. LEHMANN and D. KREBS

In an *in vitro* fertilization (IVF) programme semen analysis was carried out on 140 patients. Of these, 111 (79%) were able to fertilize at least one preovulatory oocyte *in vitro* and an embryo transfer could be performed in 90 patients. Seventeen pregnancies could be observed and to date two healthy children have been born.

Conventional parameters of semen analysis (e.g. sperm count, motility, volume, morphology) and tests of sperm function (sperm swelling test, zona free hamster ova penetration test) were performed and compared with the ability of the spermatozoa to fertilize human oocytes *in vitro*. There was only poor correlation between the fertilization rate of human sperm *in vitro* and any of the standard parameters of semen analysis (Figures 1–3).

A much better correlation could be observed between the fertilization rate and the ability of human spermatozoa to swell in a hypo-osmotic medium. The results suggest that this functional test may be useful to assess the fertilizing potential of spermatozoa and to select male patients for IVF therapy (Figure 4).

Fertilization could even be achieved in semen samples with an oligozoospermia, astenozoospermia or teratozoospermia; however, the fertilization rate of oligozoospermic samples was reduced compared with normozoospermic samples (Table 1).

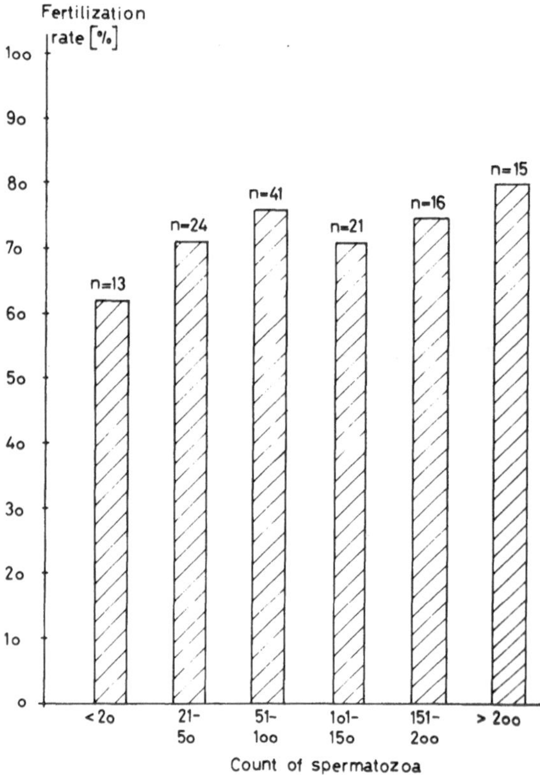

Figure 1 Fertilization rate and count of spermatozoa (in millions ml^{-1}) (n = 130)

CONCLUSIONS

(1) There is a poor correlation of standard parameters of semen analysis to fertilizing ability.

(2) There is a good correlation of 'functional tests' to fertilizing ability.

(3) 'Functional tests' may be useful in the selection of male patients for IVF.

(4) 'Swell test' is less expensive and easier to perform than 'hamster test'.

IVF and embryo transfer (ET) may have potential application in certain cases of male infertility since the close apposition of spermatozoa with preovulatory oocytes under *in vitro* conditions reduces problems of sperm transport, concentration and longevity. However, it cannot improve the quality of sperm–egg interaction. Other forms of andrological treatment should be attempted first to improve quality and quantity of spermatozoa before IVF and ET is initiated.

Table 1 Andrological diagnosis, fertilization rate and pregnancies

Diagnosis	*No. in group*	*Fertilization rate (%)*	*Pregnancies*
Normozoospermia	85	81	15
Oligozoospermia	10	60	0
Polyzoospermia	9	89	0
Asthenozoospermia	36	64	2

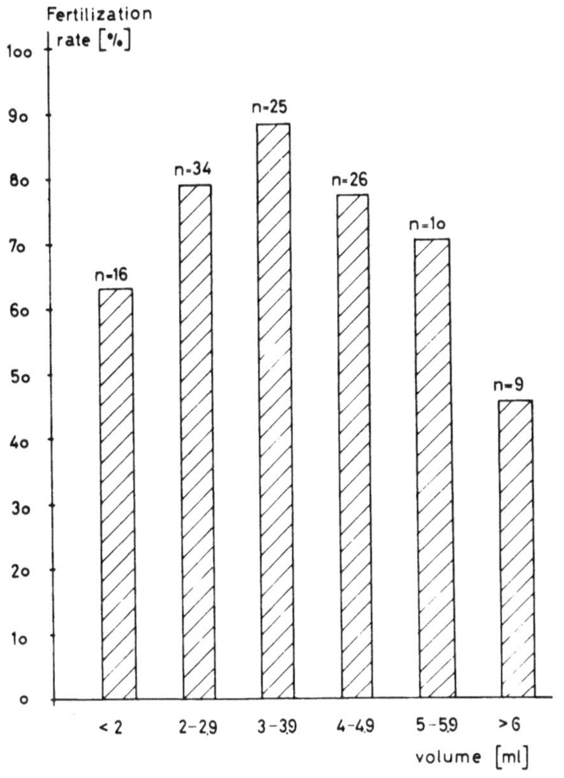

Figure 2 Fertilization rate and volume of ejaculate (in ml) ($n = 120$)

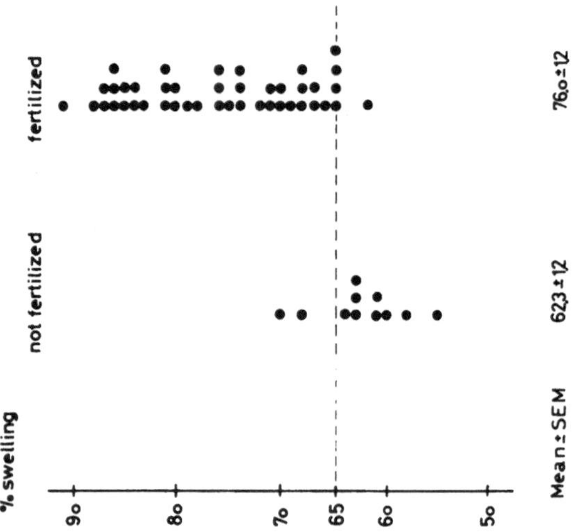

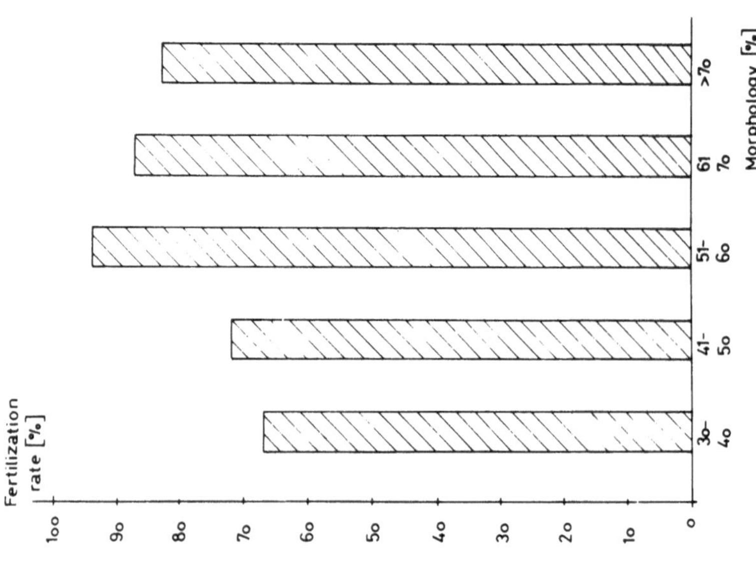

Figure 3 Fertilization rate and the morphology of spermatozoa

23
Sperm quality and *in vitro* fertilization

V. BAUKLOH, H.-H. RIEDEL, S. PAUL and L. METTLER

INTRODUCTION

Male subfertility is accepted as an indication for *in vitro* fertilization (IVF) by a number of groups[1,2]. While many groups rely merely on conventional semen analysis results for evaluating potential fertilizing capacity the problem remains as to the minimum requirements in sperm quality necessary for predicting the outcome of IVF treatment.

MATERIALS AND METHODS

Andrological categories of husbands from couples treated in the IVF programme were based on the definitions given by Schirren[4]. IVF trials were performed as described earlier[5].

In 53 cases from 1981 up to the end of 1982 bacteriological examinations were performed on the day of inseminating oocytes. A portion of the ejaculate was introduced into prefabricated media and analysed for bacterial species and the presence of T-Mycoplasma at the Hygiene Department of the University of Kiel.

RESULTS AND DISCUSSION

During the evaluation of human IVF treatments in the period from July 1982 to March 1983, 84 cases were analysed andrologically (Table 1).

Table 1 Distribution of andrological categories of semen samples from husbands whose wives were treated in the IVF programme

Group	*No. of cases*	*N*	*O*	*H*	*A*	*OA(T)*
Embryo transfer achieved	55	41 (74%)	3 (5%)	1 (2%)	2 (4%)	8 (15%)
Embryo transfer not achieved	29	19 (66%)	3 (10%)	–	1 (3%)	6 (21%)

N = Normozoospermia; O = oligozoospermia; H = hyperzoospermia; A = asthenozoospermia; T = teratozoospermia.

In 55 cases, fertilization of at least one oocyte and subsequent embryo transfer was possible while in 29 cases no fertilization occurred. The distribution of andrological categories, however, within these two groups was very similar with the portion of cases showing combined disturbed parameters being almost the same. Consistently bad fertilization results were in general only observed in samples with severe teratozoospermia or when the sperm motility decreased rapidly with time. Reduced sperm numbers or low initial motility normally were easily overcome by the IVF technique. The situation was different when fertilization rates per obtained oocyte and development of embryos were considered with regard to the andrological category of semen used for insemination (Table 2).

Table 2 Relationship between quality of semen used for insemination and cleavage rate of resulting embryos (judged after 48–50 hours)

Semen quality	*No. of oocytes inseminated*	*Unfertilized*	*2–cell stage*	*4–cell stage or beyond*
Normozoospermic	105	30 (29%)	4 (4%)	71 (67%)
One or more parameter(s) abnormal	37	19 (51%)	4 (11%)	14 (38%)

All samples with any abnormality were compiled within one group and compared with normozoospermic samples. The portion of unfertilized oocytes was definitively higher in the group with abnormal sperm parameters, while the percentage of fast-dividing embryos was clearly higher in the normozoospermic group. Nevertheless, two of the four pregnancies achieved during this period resulted after insemination of oocytes with abnormal semen (one high grade oligozoospermia, one oligo-asthenozoospermia).

The analysis of 53 cases in which a bacteriological examination was performed on the day of insemination identified 22 positive findings (42% of cases). The bacteria species found were not correlated with any of the andrological categories, with normozoospermic probes having positive bacteriology at a frequency similar to the other groups. The most common species were T-mycoplasma with 47% of all infections and enterococci with 11%. The fertilization rate of human oocytes was not affected by bacterial contaminations of the semen, but all samples producing embryos leading to pregnancy had been free of infections.

SUMMARY AND CONCLUDING REMARKS

Within the human system the influence of sperm quality was not very pronounced although the fertilization rate per obtained oocyte was lower in the group with pathological findings. Average cleavage intervals of resulting embryos appeared to be longer after insemination with sperm of abnormal parameters. Pregnancies were only obtained with fast-cleaving embryos[6]. However, two inseminations with subnormal semen samples resulted in normal pregnancies indicating that implantation was not affected. An influence of bacteria present in the semen used for insemination could not be demonstrated for fertilization although bacterial infections have been associated with infertility[7]. No pregnancy was achieved with the group with positive bacteriological findings.

Based on these results, we have established minimum sperm quality requirements for use in the IVF programme. At least two spermiocytograms must be carried out prior to the IVF trial and have (1) volumes of at least 1 ml; (2) sperm concentrations of at least 5×10^6 ml^{-1}; (3) motilities of at least 30%; and (4) percentages of sperm with normal morphology of at least 30%. Furthermore, bacteriological findings have to be negative or in cases of identified infections should be negative on two occasions after antibiotic treatment.

References

1. Trounson, A.O. and Wood, C. (1981). Extracorporeal fertilization and embryo transfer. *Clin. Obstet. Gynaecol.*, **8**, 681
2. Fishel, S.B. and Edwards, R.G. (1982). Essentials for fertilization. In Edwards, R.G. and Purdy, J.M. (eds.) *Human Conception In Vitro*. pp. 157–74. (London: Academic Press)
3. Yanagimachi, R., Yanagimachi, H. and Rogers, B.J. (1976). The use of zona free animal ova as a test system for the assessment of fertilizing capacity of human spermatozoa. *Biol. Reprod.*, **15**, 471

4. Schirren, C. (1971). *Praktische Andrologie*. (Berlin: Verlag Brüder Hartmann)
5. Mettler, L., Seki, M., Baukloh, V. and Semm, K. (1982). Human ovum recovery via operative laparoscopy and *in vitro* fertilization. *Fertil. Steril.*, **38**, 30
6. Trounson, A.O., Mohr, L.R., Wood, C. and Leeton, J.F. (1982). Effect of delayed insemination on *in vitro* fertilization, culture and transfer of human embryos. *J. Reprod. Fertil.*, **64**, 285
7. Dahlberg, B. (1976). Asymptomatic bacteriospermia – cause for infertility in men. *Urology*, **6**, 563

24
An attempt to fertilize human oocytes with epidiymal spermatozoa *in vitro*

H. VAN DER VEN, L.V. WAGENKNECHT, S. AL-HASANI, K. DIEDRICH, U. HAMERICH, F. LEHMANN, L.J.D. ZANEVELD and D. KREBS

In certain cases of transport azoospermia, e.g. due to long-distance stenosis of the vas deferens or unsuccessful reanastomosis of the vas deferens, an alloplastic spermatocele can be used to collect epididymal spermatazoa[1,2].

In this chapter we describe a patient with bilateral long-distance stenosis of the vas deferens. Spermatozoa were collected from an alloplastic spermatocele which was placed on the caput region of the epididymis as described by Wagenknecht *et al.*[2]. Because of bilateral tubal obstruction of the patient's wife, the couple attended the *in vitro* fertilization programme. To investigate the fertilizing ability of epididymal spermatozoa and importance of seminal plasma for fertilization in the human additional experiments are described using 'epididymal-like' spermatozoa[3,4].

MATERIALS AND METHODS

The human *in vitro* fertilization was basically performed as described by Lopata in 1980[5]. Briefly, the liquefied semen samples were washed twice in Ham's F10 medium, resuspended in fresh medium and the concentration was adjusted to 10–50 $\times$ 10^6 spermatozoa ml^{-1}.

The females were treated with a combination of clomiphene (days 5–9 of the cycle) and human menopausal gonadotrophin (hMG) or with clomiphene only. Ovulation was induced with an injection of human chorionic gonadotrophin (hCG) and laparoscopy and oocyte collection was performed 36 hours later.

Usually $0.1–1.0 \times 10^6$ spermatozoa were added per oocyte. Spermatozoa were separated from the oocytes after 10–20 hours and embryo transfer was performed 40–48 hours after laparoscopy. In the presented case the aspirated spermatozoa were washed twice in Ham's F10 medium immediately after collection. The female was treated with clomiphene and hMG.

The hamster oocyte penetration test was performed as described previously[6]. To obtain spermatozoa that only had minimal contact with seminal plasma ('epididymal-like' spermatozoa) a split ejaculate was performed using two jars (Figure 1). The very first fraction was ejaculated into a jar containing 200 ml BWW medium[7] without albumin and the other was empty. The highly diluted spermatozoa of the first fraction were divided into two equal portions, precipitated and resuspended in fresh BWW medium or seminal plasma that was obtained from the second fraction of the ejaculate ($2 \times 1500 \times g$, 10 min). The sperm suspensions were incubated for 20 min at a concentration of 50×10^6 sperm ml^{-1} before the hamster test was performed.

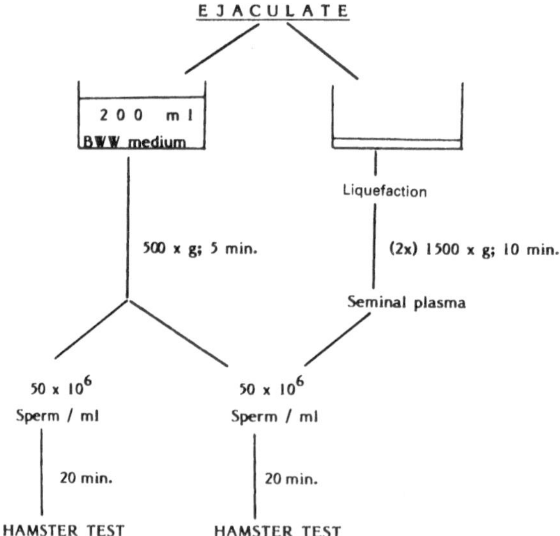

Figure 1 Effect of preincubation with homologous seminal plasma on oocyte penetration of 'epididymal-like' spermatozoa. Mean (± SE) percentage results were 50.1 ± 9 and 76.4 ± 10.7 in the samples incubated in BWW medium and those incubated in homologous seminal plasma, respectively. This difference is significant ($p < 0.05$)

RESULTS

The best aspirate (18×10^6 sperms; 20% motility) was achieved 1 week after implantation of the spermatocele (Figure 2). In the following aspirates the quality and quantity of spermatozoa decreased rapidly.

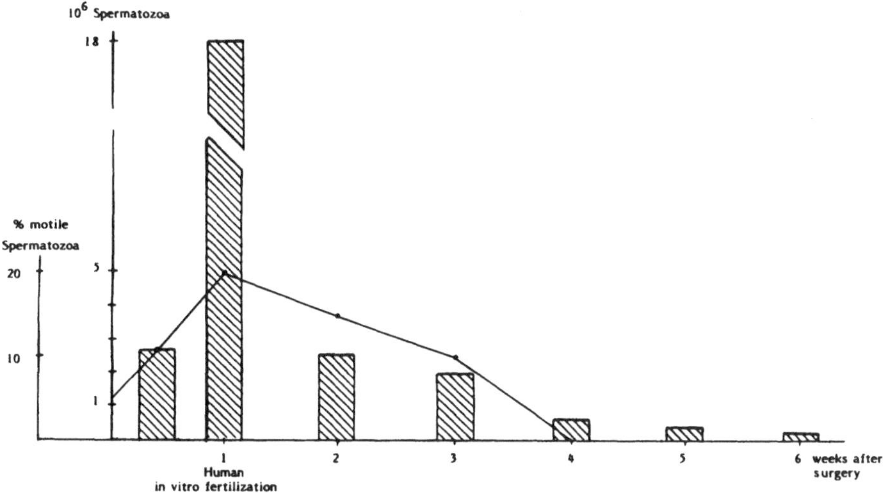

Figure 2 Results of postoperative aspirations from an alloplastic spermatocele

Out of seven oocytes that could be obtained by laparoscopic follicular puncture, five oocytes were classified to be preovulatory according to morphological criteria. However, no signs of fertilization could be observed after 48 hours in culture (Table 1). Epididymal spermatozoa could only be seen within the cumulus oopherus or on the surface of the zona pellucida. The spermatozoa were also not able to penetrate denuded hamster oocytes.

The ability of 'epididymal-like' spermatozoa to penetrate hamster oocytes was enhanced after incubation in homologous seminal plasma compared with incubation in BWW medium (76.4% and 50.1%, respectively).

DISCUSSION

A spermatocele is the only method to collect larger numbers of spermatozoa from certain infertile males. However, only a poor success

Table 1 Results of *in vitro* fertilization and hamster oocyte penetration by human epididymal spermatozoa

No. of oocytes	*Penetration of cumulus oöphorus*	*Attachment to zona pellucida*	*Signs of fertilization*
		Human in vitro fertilization	
7	Yes	Yes	No
	No. of oocytes	*Penetration (%)*	*Sperm attachment per oocyte*
		Hamster oocyte penetration	
Control	21	33	11.6
Epididymal spermatozoa:			
BWW medium	19	0	0.2
Seminal plasma	20	0	0.5

rate using these spermatozoa for artificial insemination has been reported[2,8]. A full-term delivery of a baby following insemination with spermatozoa collected from an alloplastic spermatocele was reported by Kelami[2]. In this case the aspirated spermatozoa were mixed with the ejaculate of the patient before it was used for insemination. The data presented in Figure 2 seem to support the possibility that seminal plasma contact of 'epididymal-like' and perhaps also of epididymal sperm may increase the fertilizing ability of these spermatozoa. By contrast, it is well known that human seminal plasma contains substances which inhibit fertilization[5] and Cohen *et al.*[7] could not show a beneficial effect of heterologous seminal plasma on motility and fertilizing ability of ejaculated spermatozoa. However, in a more recent study there seem to be indications of a low molecular weight penetration-enhancing factor of human seminal plasma[9]. This factor seems to be responsible for an increase in the fertilizing ability of subfertile spermatozoa and of 'epididymal-like' spermatozoa. However, in the presented case epididymal spermatozoa collected from a spermatocele did not show an enhanced penetration rate into denuded hamster oocytes following contact with donor seminal plasma.

Further studies on the fertilizing potential of human epididymal spermatozoa and on the importance of male genital tract fluids for fertilization are necessary.

CONCLUSIONS

(1) Seminal plasma may have a beneficial influence on the fertilizing capacity of human spermatozoa.

(2) The oocyte penetration rate of 'epididymal-like' spermatozoa was enhanced when spermatozoa were preincubated in their own seminal plasma.
(3) If epididymal spermatozoa or 'epididymal-like' spermatozoa (e.g. in cases of retrograde ejaculation) are used for *in vitro* fertilization or artificial insemination seminal plasma contact prior to treatment may improve the fertilizing ability

References

1. Kelami, A. (1981). Kelami–Affeld alloplastic spermatocele and successful human delivery. *Urol. Int.*, **36**, 368–72
2. Wagenknecht, L.V., Leidenberger, F.A., Schütte, B., Becker, H. and Schirren, C. (1978). Clinical experience with an alloplastic spermatocele. *Andrologie*, **10**, 417–26
3. Lindholmer, C. (1974). The importance of seminal plasma for human sperm motility. *Biol. Reprod.*, **10**, 533
4. Zaneveld, L.J.D. (1982). The epididymis. In Zaneveld, L.J.D. and Chatterton, R.T. (eds.) *Biochemistry of Mammalian Reproduction*. pp. 37–64. (New York: J. Wiley)
5. Lopata, A., Johnston, W.I.H., Hoult, I.J. and Speirs, A.L. (1980). Pregnancy following intrauterine implantation of an embryo obtained by *in vitro* fertilization of a preovulatory egg. *Fertil. Steril.*, **33**, 117–20
6. van der Ven, H., Bhattacharrya, A., Binor, Z., Leto, S. and Zaneveld, L.J.D. (1982). Inhibition of human sperm capacitation by a high molecular weight factor from human seminal plasma. *Fertil. Steril.*, **38**, 753
7. Overstreet, J.W., Yanagimachi, R., Katz, D.F., Hayashi, K. and Hanson, F.W. (1980). Penetration of human spermatozoa into the human zona pellucida and the zona free hamster egg: a study of fertile donors and infertile patients. *Fertil. Steril.*, **33**, 534
8. Cohen, J., Mooyaart, M., Vreeburg, J.T.M., Yanagimachi, R. and Zeilmaker, G.H. (1982). Fertilizing ability and motility of spermatozoa from fertile and infertile men after exposure to heterologous seminal plasma. In Hafez, E.S.E. and Semm, K. (eds.) *Instrumental Insemination*. pp. 53–62. (The Hague: Martinus Nyhoff)
9. van der Ven, H., Binor, Z. and Zaneveld, L.J.D. (1983). Beneficial effect of heterologous seminal plasma on the fertilizing capacity of human spermatozoa as assessed by the zona free hamster egg test. *Fertil. Steril.* **40**, 512

25
Infertility and sperm bacteriology

H.-H. RIEDEL, L. METTLER and K. SEMM

INTRODUCTION

Many results regarding the importance of asymptomatic bacterial infections of the female and male genital tract for fertilization *in vivo* as well as *in vitro* have been published, although very few valid conclusions can be drawn. Lately, the bacterial contamination of human sperm and female genital tract has gained special interest within the frame of *in vitro* fertilization.

In 1980 Edwards[1] pointed out that 'the bacteriology of semen should be taken very seriously' and his co-worker Webster explained that in every couple wanting to join the *in vitro* fertilization programme of the Cambridge Group, a detailed sperm examination is carried out on the husband 4–6 weeks prior to the planned treatment cycle and the semen are tested for infection prior to admitting patients into the programme.

As early as 1980, Purdy [2] and Edwards[1] required that the genital tract of a woman must be free of micro-organisms, especially of T-mycoplasma, before she can join the *in vitro* fertilization programme and that examination of the husband's ejaculate must prove the absence of pathogenic micro-organisms. Antibiotic treatment is therefore recommended if these requirements are not fulfilled by these authors, as well as by Jones[3], Feichtinger[4], Trounson[5] and other groups[6,7].

In 1977 Frazer and Taylor-Robinson[8] infected mouse oocytes and spermatozoa artifically with mycoplasma. A statistically significant reduction of *in vitro* fertilization rates was obtained associated with a significant 'reduction in embryonic development in the treated groups when compared with the untreated group'.

RESULTS

In 1982 and 1983 we started a systematic bacteriological examination of ejaculates to be used for *in vitro* fertilization.

A total of 166 ejaculates from patients taking part in the *in vitro* fertilization programme were examined. In 70 ejaculates (42.2%) bacteria concentrations greater than 10^5 ml^{-1} were found. 96 (57.8%) of the probes were negative or had bacteria concentrations less than 10^4 ml^{-1}. Mycoplasma was found in 37 (22.3%) of the examined ejaculates. The second most frequent group of micro-organisms were enterococci, found in 17 patients (10.2%). Anaerobic organisms in concentrations greater than 10^5 ml^{-1} were never detected.

When considering the sperm quality and positive, as well as negative bacteriological findings with regards to the fertilization rate of obtained oocytes the following results were obtained.

After insemination of one or more pelviscopically obtained oocytes with sperm of the husband in 16 out of 24 cases with bacteria concentrations greater than 10^5 ml^{-1} the cleavage of at least one oocyte occurred leading to an embryo transfer rate of 66.7%. Of these 16 cases in which microbiological examinations were positive, cleavage and embryo transfer of inseminated oocytes took place even though the ten cases were observed in which all inseminated oocytes were fertilized. Ten of the 16 ejaculates with positive bacteria culture but fertilizing inseminated oocytes belonged to the normozoospermic category (62.5%); only one showed a high-grade oligozoospermia. Of the eight ejaculates of the group not effecting fertilization, six (75%) were pathological and only two belonged to the normozoospermic category.

Out of 37 ejaculates with negative bacteriological finding, 19 (51.4%) fertilized at least one of the inseminated oocytes. Of these 19 ejaculates, 11 (57.9%) belonged to the normozoospermic category while the remainder showed a more or less clear pathospermy.

Of the 18 bacteriologically negative ejaculates not fertilizing the obtained oocytes only seven (38.9%) belonged to the normozoospermic category, while 12 were clearly pathological. Of the 19 ejaculates of this group fertilizing at least one of the pelviscopically obtained oocytes, 11 (57.1%) succeeded in fertilizing all obtained oocytes.

DISCUSSION

From the results obtained up to now any direct effect of micro-organism-contaminated sperm on the human *in vitro* fertilization system resulting in reduced fertilization rates cannot be demonstrated. The cleavage and embryo transfer rates within the group with positive bacteriological findings in the sperm were even higher than within the group with negative bacteriological findings. But the 21 pregnancies we obtained all resulted from bacteria-free sperm.

In our examinated collective no statistically significant correlations between positive or negative bacteriological findings and the andrological category and cytology of the ejaculate smears were found. Remarkably, no correlation existed between the so-called 'leukocytospermy' and positive bacteriological findings. In four cases of severe leukocytospermy several sperm checks always showed negative microbiological test results.

The possibility that groups of bacteria not always detectable during routine andrological diagnosis – as for example certain species of anaerobic organisms – may be perhaps responsible for the occurrence of these leukocytospermy cannot totally be excluded since pertinent data are also not available from the literature[9].

No correlation existed between special groups of bacteria andrological diagnosis and differential spermiocytograms. The most common germs detected by microbiological examinations – such as T-Mycoplasma and enterococci – were found in ejaculates of the normozoospermic category, as well as in pathological ejaculates, and these were not associated with specific cytological changes. We are therefore unable to confirm the correlation reported by Derrick and Dahlberg[10] between increasing leukocyte concentrations and decreasing sperm quality, which was used to explain the interrelation between infections of the male genital tract and reduced fertility rates.

The existence of leukocytes or of leukocytospermy within the ejaculate is not correlated with special inflammations of the male genital tract. Likewise a statistically justified relationship between reduced fertili-zation and the occurrence of certain species of bacteria within the ejaculate was not found. Even in leukocyte-free ejaculate concentrations of micro-organisms greater than 10^5 ml^{-1} were demonstrated and leukocytospermy was detectable with negative bacteriological findings.

In conclusion, it can be said that there is no relation between microbiological and cytological findings of ejaculates used for insemination of oocytes and the obtained fertilization-, cleavage- and embryo transfer rates in the human *in vitro* fertilization programme here. But since a negative effect on implantation rates or embryonic development cannot be excluded, detailed bacteriological examinations and probably antibiotic treatment may be recommended before admission into an *in vitro* fertilization programme.

References

1. Edwards, R.G. and Steptoe, P.C. (1980). Establishing fullterm human pregnancies using cleaving embryos grown *in vitro*. *Br. J. Obstet. Gynaecol.*, **87**, 737-56
2. Purdy, J.M. (1980). Pregnancies with embryos grown *in vitro*. *Br. J. Obstet. Gynaecol.*, **87**, 757–768
3. Jones, H. (1982). Discussion on the fertilization of human oocytes *in vivo* and *in vitro*. In Edwards, R.G. and Purdy, J.M. (eds.) *Human Conception in Vitro*. pp. 191-200 (New York: Academic Press)
4. Feichtinger, W., Szalay, S., Kemeter, P., Beck, A. and Janish, H. (1981). *In vitro* Fertilisierung menschlicher Eizellen sowie Embryotransfer. *Geburtsh. Frauenheilkd.*, **41**, 482-89
5. Trounson, A.O. (1982). Factors influencing the success of fertilization and embryonic growth *in vitro*. In Edwards, R.G. and Purdy, J.M. (eds.) *Human Conception in Vitro*. pp. 201-207 (New York: Academic Press)
6. Fishel, S.B. and Edwards, R.G. (1982). Essential of fertilization. In Edwards, R.G. and Purdy, J.M. (eds.) *Human Conception In Vitro*. pp. 157–74 (New York: Academic Press)
7. Purdy, J.M. (1982). Methods for fertilization and embryo culture *in vitro*. In Edwards, R.G. and Purdy, J.M. (eds.) *Human Conception in Vitro*. pp. 135–56. (New York: Academic Press)
8. Frazer, L. and Taylor-Robinson, D. (1977). The effect of mycoplasma pulmonis on fertilization and preimplantation development *in vitro* of mouse eggs. *Fertil. Steril.*, **28**, 488-98
9. Riedel, H.-H. (1980). Techniques for the detection of leucocytospermia in human semen. *Arch. Androl.*, **5**, 287–93

Part IV

In vitro Fertilization and Embryo Transfer. Clinical Results

Part IV

Section 1
In Humans

26
Course of pregnancy and delivery after *in vitro* fertilization and embryo transfer

S. SZALAY, F. FISCHL, E. MÜLLER-TYL and H. JANISCH

On the 5th of August 1982 the first baby to be born in Austria after *in vitro* fertilization and embryo transfer (IVF and ET) was delivered at the 2nd Department of Gynaecology and Obstetrics of the University of Vienna. He was healthy, weighed 3650 g and was 52 cm long. The course of pregnancy and delivery had been without complications.

In the meantime, in the same department, a total number of 25 pregnancies were achieved and 12 babies born. One of these was a twin delivery.

The average age of the patients was 29 years; the youngest was 21 years old and the oldest 38. The average pregnancy rate per transfer, according to all performed transfers, was 17% (single transfer, 11%; double transfer, 23%, triple transfer, 24%). It is also very interesting that more than two-thirds of all pregnancies occurred after the first ET (18 pregnancies after first transfer, six after second transfer, one after third transfer). Of these 25 pregnancies, eight patients (32%) aborted in the 6th to 13th week of gestation. Twice an ectopic pregnancy was seen. Until now a total of four twin pregnancies were achieved. The course of pregnancies of the patients who have delivered was without any major complications (Table 1). The average increase of weight during the pregnancy was 13.5 kg. The values of the blood pressure were in all patients within the normal range. Oedema was seen only in one case

Table 1 Course of pregnancies after *in vitro* fertilization

Patient	*Weight gain(kg)*	*RR*	*Oedema*	*Proteinuria*
1	22	–	+	–
2	13	–	–	–
3	11	–	–	–
4	11	–	+	–
5	15	–	+	–
6	12	–	+	+
7	11	–	–	–
8	13	–	–	–
9	11	–	+	–
10	7	–	–	–
11	20	–	+++	–

(twin pregnancy). Albuminuria was in all cases negative. Only in one patient was there a transient albuminuria at the end of pregnancy. The average duration of delivery was about 7 hours. The mode of delivery was spontaneous in four cases; in three patients a delivery by forceps was performed and in four patients a caesarean section was done (Table 2).

Table 2 Mode of delivery in pregnancies after *in vitro* fertilization

Patient	*Mode of delivery*	*Indication*
1	Sectio	Protracted delivery
2	Forceps	i.u. asphyxia
3	Spontaneous	–
4	Forceps	Diminished contractions
5	Sectio	i.u. asphyxia
6	Forceps	Diminished contractions
7	Spontaneous	–
8	Spontaneous	–
9	Spontaneous	–
10	Sectio	i.u. asphyxia
11	Sectio	gemini, prematurity

The average birth weight – exluding the twins – was 3215 g (Table 3) (2250–3700 g). The average length was 50 cm. The paediatric development of all children so far is completely normal. In conclusion one can say, that the method of IVF and ET is now fully established as a routine method in this department and can be offered as a treatment for certain sterility problems.

Table 3 Birth weights and length in pregnancies after *in vitro* fertilization

Patient	*Sex*	*Birth weight(g)*	*Length(cm)*
1	M	3700	53
2	F	3000	50
3	F	3600	51
4	M	3650	52
5	M	2250	46
6	F	3400	51
7	M	2800	45
8	F	3500	53
9	F	2950	47
10	M	3300	51
11	F/F	2200/2400	42/44

27
Successful *in vitro* fertilization: practical technique and first results with cryo-sperma. Fertility Centre – Vienna

P. HERNUSS

Since January 1983, our Fertility Centre has offered the possibility of treating sterile couples with the means of *in vitro* fertilization and embryo transfer (IVF and ET).

Up to April 2nd, 25 patients were laparoscopied after stimulation with clomiphene and hCG (choriongonadotrophin) to recover oocytes. In 14 patients at least one oocyte could be found. This corresponds to a rate of oocyte removal of 88%. In total, 30 mature oocytes were recovered.

The technique of egg culture is performed corresponding to the successfully used method of the 'II. Universitäts-Frauenklinik', Vienna. This consists of maturation of the oocyte in the medium (Inra-Menezo B2) after adding 75% of follicular fluid, transfer into the fertilizing medium (B^{II}), insemination 41 hours after application of hCG with 100 000–200 000 sperms, evaluation of a correct fertilization 18–20 hours afterwards and transfer into the growth medium (B^{II} + serum).

Fertilization was achieved in 15 patients; a fertilization rate of 60% could therefore be reached. The following circumstances were responsible for unsuccessful fertilization: oliogasthenospermia in two patients, infection of the sperms despite prophylactic administration of antibiotics in two patients and an agglutination of fibrin remaining in the serum in one patient.

In 11 patients, ET was performed, which corresponds to a transfer rate of 44% for all patients and a cleavage rate of 73%. Up to April 2nd, 1983, the success of six transfers was evaluated. Two pregnancies were manifested, proved by hCG specification in the serum and LH specification in the urine and in the serum. Heart activity was confirmed with ultrasound in one patient. For fertilization, cryo-sperma was used in eight of the patients.

28
Pregnancy after *in vitro* fertilization and embryo transfer in Singapore

S.C. NG, S.S. RATNAM, H.Y. LAW, M. RAUFF, P.C. WONG, C.M. CHIA, H.H.V. GOH, C. ANANDAKUMAR, K.E. LEONG and S.C. YEOH

INTRODUCTION

In vitro fertilization and embryo transfer (IVF and ET) is becoming an important technique in the treatment of subfertility. It is the method of choice in irreversibly damaged Fallopian tubes, and is gaining widespread use in oligospermia and idiopathic subfertility.

In Singapore, the Ovum Culture Laboratory was started in December 1981. This came about after a member of the team was sent to Monash University, Melbourne, in June 1981 for 4 weeks under the supervision of Alan Trounson. The initial 6 months were occupied with murine experiments. It was only when we were able to obtain cleavage of murine ova fertilized *in vitro* to two cells of between 80 and 100% that we attempted IVF and ET in women.

This was in July 1982. The first patient was a 29-year-old Chinese patient who had bilateral tubal damage. She had three follicles on clomiphene (Clomid) stimulation. However, the laparoscopic recovery of ova was unsuccessful, perhaps because we had to rotate the only two Falcon test tubes we had throughout the operation. The second patient suffered from irreversible tubal occlusion, and had only one follicle following Clomid. Her laparoscopy was timed 25 hours from the onset of spontaneous LH surge; however, it was too late as ovulation had occurred spontaneously. The third patient was a 30-year-old Indian who had a previous salpingectomy for an ectopic pregnancy, and the remaining tube was hypoplastic. An ovum was recovered from a single follicle following Clomid, and after fertilization developed to eight cells in 59 hours. However, the ET was difficult and no pregnancy ensued.

THE PATIENT

The fourth patient was a 25-year-old Chinese who had 4 years of primary subfertility due to bilateral cornual obstruction of the Fallopian tubes. Her last menstrual period was on 28 August 1982. Clomid 50 mg three times daily was taken from day 2 for five days. On her 10th day, ultrasound revealed a follicle 1.1 × 1.1 × 1.1 cm on her right ovary. This grew to 1.4 × 1.6 × 1.6 cm on day 12 when she was admitted, and to 1.9 × 2.5 × 1.8 cm on day 15 with a cumulus oophorus measuring 0.7 cm. Her serum oestradiol-17β measured 232 pg ml^{-1} on day 10, and increased to 1085 pg ml^{-1} on day 14 (Table 1). Three-hourly urine measurements of LH by Higonavis from day 12 showed no spontaneous surge. Intramuscular Pregnyl 5000 IU was given on day 15 and the laparoscopic recovery timed 30 hours later. A single preovulatory follicle measuring 2.5 cm in diameter was seen and aspirated. A preovulatory ovum was obtained.

Table 1 Follicular growth as indicated by ultrasound and serum oestradiol level

Day of cycle	*Serum oestradiol (pg ml^{-1})*	*Follicular volume (ml)*
10	232	0.70
11	408	1.33
12	396	1.88
13	795	2.27
14	1085	2.67
15	1152	4.48
16	1073	2.26

FERTILIZATION AND GROWTH

The ovum was matured for a further 6 hours in 0.5 ml of T6 medium with 10% heat-deactivated human serum and 0.5 ml follicular fluid before insemination. The semen was collected 2 hours before insemination, washed with medium, centrifuged at 500 rpm for 10 minutes and layered with 0.5 ml medium. After 30 minutes the supernatant was collected. Half a million treated spermatozoa in 27 μl were then introduced into the Falcon tube with the ovum. After 17.5 hours two pronuclei were seen. Growth times were within those reported by Edwards *et al.*[1] (Table 2).

Table 2 Stages of fertilization and growth *in vitro*

Stage	*Time from insemination (hr)*	*Expected time (hr)*
2 pronuclei	17.5	–
3 blastomeres	34.75	–
4 blastomeres	46.0	49.0 ± 1.3

From reference 1.

EMBRYO TRANSFER

The four-cell embryo was transferred using the method described by Leeton *et al.*[2]. The catheter used was a Monash Embryo Transfer Set I (William A. Cook Australia Pty Ltd). The transfer was effected in the lithotomy position without any anaesthesia and any difficulty. The volume of medium transferred with the embryo was 20 μl.

POST-REPLACEMENT REGIMEN

The patient was placed on complete rest in bed in the supine position for 24 hours. Depo Proluton (17-OH progesterone caproate, Schering AG) was administered: 250 mg on POD1 (1st day after laparoscopy), 500 mg on POD2, POD3, POD5 and subsequently twice a week from POD12. Her hCG level showed a rise by the 11th POD (9th day after ER)(Table 3). Ultrasound showed a gestational sac on the 23rd POD, measuring 5 × 5 × 4 mm.

Her pregnancy progressed satisfactorily. Ultrasound biparietal diameters were within acceptable limits (Figure 1), while 24-hour urinary oestriols were satisfactory. Antenatal CTGs from 32 weeks' gestation were reactive. Labour was surgically induced on 19th May 1983, at the beginning of the 38th week of gestation, and delivery was by forceps 7.5 hours later. The healthy male infant, weighing 2535 g, was without any obvious congenital defects.

Table 3 Oestradiol, progesterone and human chorionic gonadotrophin (hCG) values following laparoscopy

Days after laparoscopy	*Oestradiol* ($pg\ ml^{-1}$)	*Progesterone* ($ng\ ml^{-1}$)	*hCG* ($mIU\ ml^{-1}$)
5	387	23.6	10.3
8	281	21.0	4.9
11	416	28.9	>500
14	804	36.9	>500
17	518	30.8	>500
20	935	41.2	>500

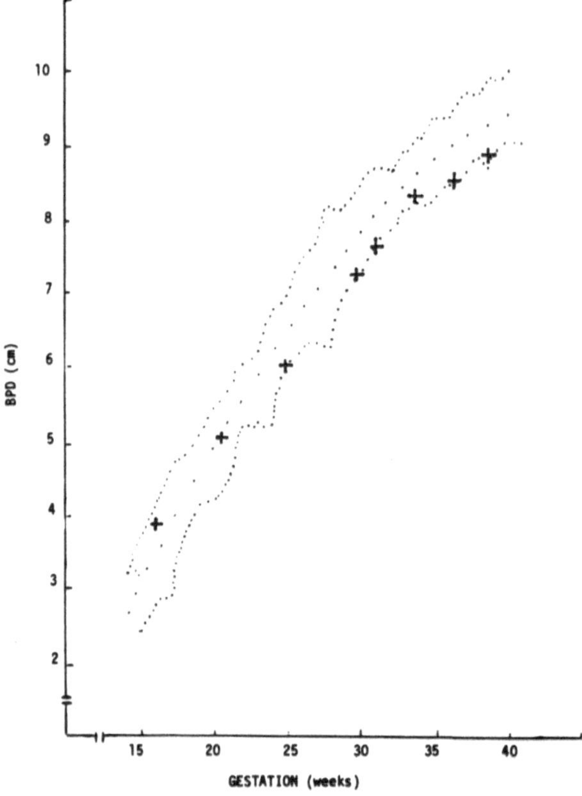

Figure 1 Ultrasound biparietal diameters (BPD) during gestation

DISCUSSION

At the time of writing (May 1983), we have done 20 laparoscopies on 26 patient-cycles, recovered 12 ova from 11 patients, fertilized and cleaved nine of the ova, replaced nine embryos in eight patients, and achieved one pregnancy. Our success rate is much lower than reported rates[3,4]. However, there were three couples who had oligospermia and four couples with idiopathic subfertility, and such problems signify poorer pregnancy rates[3].

Progesterone support in the luteal phase is controversial. Work with primates suggests compromised progesterone production in a third of them[5]. However, clinical studies have not been convincing[6,7]. Yovich *et al.* have reported the use of oral medroxyprogesterone acetate[8]. We have used high doses of parental 17OH-progesterone caproate but we have not continued with it.

Acknowledgements

We wish to thank the Ministry of Health, Singapore, for allowing us to undertake this project, the National University of Singapore for the financial and related support, and the staff and nurses in Kandang Kerbau Hospital who have assisted in making this project a success.

References

1. Edwards, R.G., Purdy, J.M., Steptoe, P.C. and Walters, D.E. (1981). The growth of human pre-implantation embryos *in vitro*. *Am. J. Obstet. Gynecol.*, **141**, 408–16
2. Leeton, J., Trounson, A., Jessup, D. and Wood, C. (1982). The techniques for human embryo transfer. *Fertil. Steril.*, **38**, 156–61
3. Trounson, A.O. and Wood, C. (1981). Extracorporeal fertilization and embryo transfer. *Clin. Obstet. Gynecol.*, **8**, 681–713
4. Steptoe, P.C. (1982). Test-tube babies. Plenary lecture presented at the *16th Singapore-Malaysia Congress of Medicine*. 19–23 July 1982, Singapore
5. Kreitman, O., Nixon, W.E. and Hodgen, G.D. (1981). Induced corpus luteum dysfuction after aspiration of the preovulatory follicle in monkeys. *Fertil. Steril.*, **35**, 671–5
6. Feichtinger, W., Kemeter, P., Szalay, S., Beck, A. and Janisch, H. (1982). Could aspiration of the Graafian follicle cause luteal phase deficiency? *Fertil. Steril.*, **37**, 205–8.
7. Garcia, J., Jones, G.S., Acosta, A.A. and Wright, G.L. (1981). Corpus luteum function after follicle aspiration for oocyte retrieval. *Fertil. Steril.*, **36**, 565–72
8. Yovich, J., Puzey, A., de'Atta, R., Roberts, R., Reid, S. and Grauaug, A. (1982). *In-vitro* fertilization pregnancy with early progestagen support. *Lancet*, **2**, 378–9

29
In vitro fertilization and embryo transfer: an out-patient procedure?

J.T. HAZEKAMP, P. FYLLING and A. HØISETH

Significant developments have occurred in the field of *in vitro* fertilization and embryo transfer (IVF and ET) in humans since the momentous success of Edwards and Steptoe in 1978[1]. Trounson from the Monash group in Melbourne at the Third Congress of Human Reproduction in West Berlin during March 1981 elegantly showed the advantages of using stimulated cycles[2], a method previously placed in disrepute[3], and at the Reinier De Graaf conference in Nijmegen during the same year, Suzan Lenz from the Copenhagen group virtually placed IVF and ET straight into the polyclinic with her lecture on ultrasound-guided follicle aspiration[4]. At the 39th Annual Meeting of the American Fertility Society the Norfolk group opened wider the aspiration window when they reported two pregnancies (one of them concluded) after *in vitro* oocyte maturation[5].

At Ullevaal Hospital we have been constantly aware of the potential for Out-patient IVF therapy and abandoned laparoscopic oocyte retrieval for an ultrasound-guided method in October 1982.

This is a presentation of our first 70 attempts in 53 infertile couples, mostly with severe tubal infertility (90%).

Stimulated cycles were used in all cases, most of the patients being treated with clomiphene citrate (Clomivid, Draco) 100 mg daily from day 5 to day 9. All patients were given an intramuscular injection of human chorionic gonadotrophin (hCG)(Physex, Leo) 4500 IE approximately 35 hours before a scheduled follicle aspiration.

FOLLICLE MONITORING

Follicles were monitored by ultrasound only. Daily examinations were started on the 10th day of the treatment cycle. Patients were instructed to attend the clinic with a full bladder. They were requested to refrain from micturition for 3 hours before the examination and to drink half a litre of fluid during this period.

Follicles were measured in three planes and average diameter of the dominant follicle was calculated. The cumulus mass was observed as suggested by the Copenhagen group[6]. The injection of hCG was given during the early hours of the day after a follicle diameter of 20 mm or more was registered. Although hormone tests were also done, results were available only in retrospect for individual case analysis.

FOLLICLE ASPIRATION

The majority of aspirations were done on the 14th or 15th day of the cycle according to our regimen, and these aspirations also provided the best results. Oocyte retrieval was best on day 15 (1.4 oocytes per patient) while oocytes collected on day 14 provided the best cleavage rate (57.1%). The difference, however, is not significant. A Philips SDR 2000 Real-time Sector scanner with 3.5 MHz to 5 MHz sound head was used for monitoring follicles and the follicle aspirations. A video-recording was made of several aspirations enabling review of aspiration difficulties.

Patients were not hospitalized for follicle aspiration. They arrived 1 hour in advance and returned home 1 hour after the procedure. Patients were allowed a normal breakfast on aspiration day. Aspirations were usually scheduled for 13.00. Immediately on arrival the patient was given an oral dose of diazepam 10 mg (Vival, A-L). She was placed on a comfortable examination bench for relaxing. 20 minutes before aspiration the bladder was emptied with a catheter and refilled with 300–600 ml of Ringers Lactate solution pre-warmed to 37°C. Follicles were located by ultrasound and measured. The pre-vesicle abdominal wall was infiltrated with local anaesthesia, lidocain HC1 0.5% (Xylocain, Astra). 10 minutes before the procedure the patient was given 100 mg Petidine by intravenous injection.

A siliconized (Sigmacote, Sigma Chemical Company) metal cannula with internal diameter 1.3 mm and external diameter 1.5 mm was used for the aspirations. The tip of the needle was machined to procure better ultrasound visibility, similarly to the needles used in Gothenborg for the same purpose[7]. There was no stylet in the needle. Suction pressure was 100 mmH_2O.

We have designed an ultrasound head attachment specifically to facilitate puncture of ovarian follicles, and have used it with apparent benefit in the later part of our series. The attachment allows for cannula mobility within the ultrasound plane. Puncture of follicles is possible when they are best demonstrated on the ultrasound screen, and at right angles to the follicle wall in closest proximity to the bladder.

Oocytes are located under an operating microscope with a zoom lens and underneath light source. Insemination was usually done 5–6 hours after oocyte retrieval. A semen specimen was collected only after a positive oocyte find. A modified T6 medium (Whittingham) was used containing 8% (pre-hCG) human serum in the fertilization medium and 15% serum in the embryo culture medium.

Transcervical embryo transfer was usually done at 45–55 hours, at the 4-cell stage. Catheter methods and types were changed several times during this series. A few embryos were transferred a day later at the 8-cell stage. Patients received no medication before transfer. They were kept in bed for 10–18 hours following transfer, overnight if the transfer was performed during the evening. The role of bed rest after embryo transfer is probably empiric and likely to disappear from the regimen.

RESULTS

Table 1 IVF and ET results

	No. (%) of patients
Failed aspiration	23 (32.9)
Oocytes collected	47 (67.1)
Cleavage	32 (45.7)
Transfer	29 (41.4)
Fertilization rate (out of 72 oocytes)	42 (58.3)
Transfer rate (out of 72 oocytes)	38 (52.7)
Pregnancies:	1 tubal pregnancy

Results have been both encouraging and discouraging (Table 1). Oocyte retrieval, cleavage rate and transfer rate are acceptable at this early stage in our work even though it cannot yet concur with the best laparoscopic oocyte retrieval results. With an oocyte retrieval of approximately one per patient it is not surprising that the cleavage rate is not higher. It is not always the best oocyte that ends up in the culture dish. As the aspiration technique improves and more oocytes become available cleavage rate can be expected to improve.

The disappointment lies in the low implantation rate. Only one pregnancy resulted after 29 embryo transfers, and unhappily this implantation occurred in the tube. The diagnosis was confirmed by serum hCG tests (over 6000 units) and on laparoscopy. So-called chemical pregnancies have been excluded. Follicle growth was similar for the cleavage (transfer) group when compared with growth of follicles in the non-cleavage group (Figure 1).

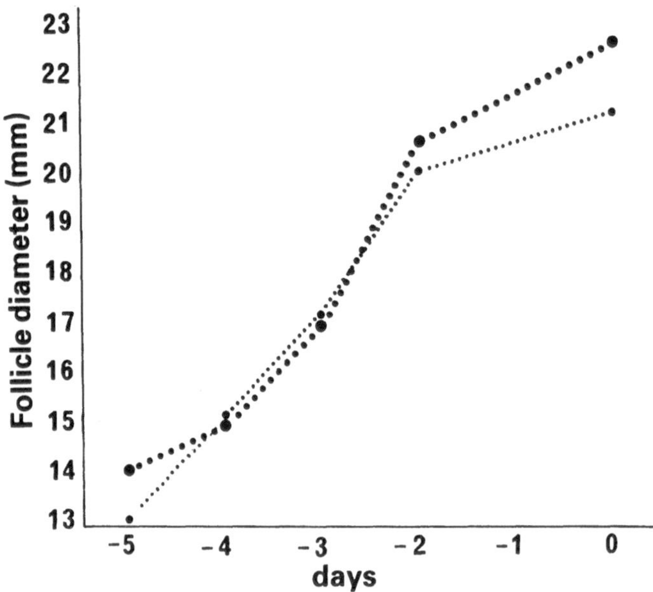

Figure 1 Ultrasound follicle monitoring in 28 oocyte cleavage cycles (bold circles) and 13 no-cleavage cycles (faint circles)

Our mentors in IVF and ET in England and Australia have been slow to utilize ultrasound for follicle puncture despite a great deal of experience with ultrasound follicle monitoring[8], and Edwards has expressed some reservations on the role of ultrasound in IVF[9]. In

Scandinavia we find this difficult to understand. The benefits of ultrasound aspiration and monitoring are clear. The procedure is relatively simple and readily repeatable in patients who must often go through many treatment cycles before achieving a pregnancy. There is a cost reduction both relative to staff requirements and hormone analysis. With a lower staff requirement planning is also simplified.

The procedure excludes potentially toxic intraperitoneal gas[10]. Adherences which exclude the laparoscopic method usually present no difficulty for the ultrasound technique. We have not observed any complications after these 70 transvesicle oocyte aspirations and no complications have been reported by the groups in Copenhagen and Gothenborg. The technique was well tolerated in 75% of the attempts. In only 3% did the patients experience unacceptable pain.

We believe development in ultrasound techniques to be of major importance to reduce cost and increase availability of IVF and ET.

References

1. Edwards, R.G., Steptoe, P.C. and Purdy, J.M. (1980). Establishing full term human pregnancies using cleaving embryos grown *in vitro*. *Br. J. Obstet. Gynaecol.*, **87**, 757
2. Trounson, A.O. *et al.* (1981). Successful *in vitro* fertilization and embryo transfer in the controlled ovulatory cycle. Presented at the *III World Congress of Human Reproduction*, March 22–26, Berlin
3. Edwards, R.G. (1980). Back to nature. In Edwards, R.G. and Steptoe, P.C. (eds.) *A Matter of Life*. pp. 134–40. (London: Hutchinson)
4. Lenz, S. and Lauritsen, J.G. (1982). Ultrasonically guided percutaneous aspiration of human follicles under local anaesthesia: a new method of collecting oocytes for *in vitro* fertilization. *Fertil. Steril.*, **39**, 458
5. Veeck, L.L., Wortham, J.R. and Jones, H.W. (1983). Maturation and fertilization of human oocytes in a program of *in vitro* fertilization. *Fertil. Steril.*, **39**, 437
6. Lauritsen, J.G. (1983). Paper presented at the *Nordic Meeting on In Vitro Fertilization*, April 14–17, Bardola
7. Wikland, M., *et al.* (1983). Collection of human oocytes by the use of sonography. (In preparation)
8. Buttery, B., *et al.* (1983). Evaluation of diagnostic ultrasound as a parameter of follicular development in an *in vitro* fertilization program. *Fertil. Steril.*, **39**, 458
9. Edwards, R.G. (1982). Effect of the gas phase on oocytes during difficult laparoscopies. In Edwards, R.G. and Purdy, J.M. (eds.) *Human Conception In Vitro*. p. 122. (London: Academic Press)
10. Edwards, R.G. (1982). Does ultrasound influence the time of ovulation. In Edwards, R.G. and Purdy, J.M. (eds.) *Human Conception In Vitro*. pp. 85–95. (London: Academic Press)

30
Current status of human *in vitro* fertilization

R.G. EDWARDS

The situation today concerning human fertilization *in vitro* has been transformed beyond recognition. From the early, challenging ideas of 1965 the clinical opportunities of the method were first demonstrated in 1975, when the first embryo implanted after replacement in the uterus; unfortunately, this turned out to be an ectopic pregnancy. 2 years later, the birth of the first children conceived through *in vitro* fertilization (IVF) ushered in the beginnings of this new form of clinical medicine for the alleviation of infertility and, perhaps, for the avoidance of inherited disorders by identifying embryos which were afflicted with genetic disorders. Today, the potential of IVF as the cure for infertility has been amply proven, as I hope to show below.

Several steps in the procedure had to be solved before it became a clinical treatment. Most aspects of the work are now under a large measure of control. There is no difficulty in persuading one or more follicles to grow in the ovary, by the use of treatments such as clomiphene, human menopausal gonadotrophin (hMG), tamoxifen or combinations of these methods. Indeed, several oocytes have been collected from ovaries since 1970, when mild forms of superovulation in cyclic women were introduced[1]. Different clinics now use various methods most suited to their own requirements, and have developed monitoring systems enabling them to assess follicular growth by ultrasound or by endocrine measurements. It is not difficult to induce the growth of several follicles in a patient, and many will ovulate in response to an endogenous LH surge or to an injection of human chorionic gonadotrophin (hCG). Moreover, simpler methods of aspirating oocytes are being introduced. This was first suggested by Lentz and Lauritsen in 1982[2] and by Wikland and his associates[3], and excellent progress in the ultrasonic aspiration of oocytes has been reported recently by several groups of workers[4]. This method promises to avoid the need for general anaesthesia for many patients, to simplify the whole procedure for aspirating oocytes and to open new non-invasive methods of examining follicles and other internal organs. Laparoscopy is still the most widely used method for collecting oocytes, with very high levels of success. Some indication of the incidence of success with these methods is provided in a recent series of 150 patients in Bourn Hall; one or more preovulatory oocytes were collected from 96% of them, and the proportion of oocytes from individual follicles approached 90%. Other clinics have reported similar success rates, and it is clear that the endocrine and surgical methods for aspirating oocytes are becoming simplified and routine.

There is, however, at least one reservation about these treatments used to stimulate ovulation. We do not know enough about the nature of growth of individual follicles, especially under conditions of heavy superovulation. The only measure to assess growth is by ultrasound, which measures the size of a follicle, but this is not enough. The largest follicle is not necessarily the most advanced, and smaller follicles may be preovulatory[1,5]. It was clear some years ago that there was some variation in the degree of maturation amongst the several follicles responding to human menopausal gonadotrophins[6], implying that some follicles are more mature than others. This observation was based on the varying steroid concentrations in different follicles. Perhaps such variations are unimportant endocrinologically, because the dominant or leading follicles may be able to sustain an adequate luteal phase and a pregnancy. On the other hand, the luteinization of several follicles, resulting in high levels of plasma progesterone in the luteal phase, may lead to disorders in uterine development, and this point has not been satisfactorily established in any clinic as far as I am aware.

Another, perhaps more important consideration arises from the growth of several follicles. Since follicles vary in their developmental maturation, it is also possible that the oocytes also vary in their potential. An arbitrarily timed injection of hCG could induce some oocytes to mature before they were fully competent to do so, e.g. before they had fully completed their preovulatory synthesis of proteins. The incidence of fertilization, the growth of embryos *in vitro,* and – most important – the incidence of implantation could therefore vary among oocytes collected from follicles in different stages of growth, and this may be reflected in poor performance results for IVF as a whole. There is, indeed, clear evidence from our own work that the occurrence of a natural LH surge after treatment with clomiphene gives higher rates of pregnancy than does treatment with clomiphene and injection of hCG (Table 1). The reason could well be that the dominant follicle causes the LH surge and also produces an embryo which is capable of implanting more successfully than are oocytes produced in response to hCG. The hCG is administered at a convenient time to perform subsequent laparoscopy, and not because of any clear indication that follicles are ready to ovulate; its use in such an arbitrary manner may be 'paid for' by a lower rate of implantation. We therefore make great efforts to permit the LH surge to occur, and to monitor it very carefully; hCG is given only when oestrogen levels are very high, large (> 2.0 cm) follicles are present, and the LH surge has not begun. Laparoscopy for oocyte recovery is then carried out 26 h after the first rising assay for urinary LH, or 34–36 h after an injection of hCG.

There can also be little doubt that fertilization and embryonic growth *in vitro* are under a high degree of control in many clinics. On our experience, the rates of fertilization are very high (over 90%), provided the samples of semen contain progressively motile spermatozoa, and are free of antibodies, inflammatory cells or debris (Table 2). Under such circumstances, more than 90% of oocytes are fertilized, and more than 95% of the subsequent embryos are replaced in the mother. Such levels of success are so high that rare variations in spermatozoa such as ultrastructural or biochemical defects, or the aspiration of a few incompletely matured oocytes, could explain the failure rate. The media used are very simple: Earle's solution with pyruvate, penicillin and the patient's own inactivated serum. It would be difficult to find a simpler medium, yet it sustains the growth of embryos until blastocysts[8]. Some clearly obvious conditions in semen reduce fertilization rates drastically: antibodies causing slumping of the spermatozoa, inflammatory damage resulting in numerous leukocytes and other cells in the semen, large amounts of debris of unknown origin, and inadequate forward movement of spermatozoa. These problems offer a major area for research in methods to improve success rates for patients with these afflictions. We believe that studies on the male could result in the alleviation of a great deal of infertility and stress for those couples.

Many unusual observations have been made on fertilization and embryonic growth *in vitro*. Increasingly, it is becoming apparent that the final stages of oocyte maturation can be completed *in vitro*, and that many pregnancies can result. In Bourn Hall, we must sometimes

Table 1 Clinical pregnancies in relation to the treatment and the number of embryos replaced[7].

No. of embryos replaced	*Natural cycle*		*Clomiphene/LH surge*		*Clomiphene/hCG*		*Other stimulants*	
	No. of patients	*No. (%) pregnant*	*No. of patients*	*No. (%) pregnant*	*No. of patients*	*No. (%) pregnant*	*No. of patients*	*No. (%) pregnant*
One	250	38 (15.2)	228	37 (16.2)	109	13 (11.9)	31	4 (12.8)
Two	7	1 (14.3)	111	34 (30.6)	111	25 (22.5)	10	3 (30.0)
Three			8	3 (37.5)	15	2 (13.3)	10	2 (20.0)
Four					1	1		

The binomial expansion for clomiphene/LH surge, where $a = 0.16$, predicts 33 pregnancies when two embryos are replaced, and 3.3 after replacing three. With clomiphene/hCG, where $a = 0.12$, 24.9 pregnancies would be expected with two embryos and 4.8 with three.

Table 2 Incidence of fertilization *in vitro*

Spermatozoa	*Total no. of patients*	*No. (%) with one oocyte fertilized*	*Oocytes fertilized (%)*
Influence of various conditions in semen			
Satisfactory	95	87 (92)	85
Head clumps, viscous seminal plasma	11	10 (90)	95
Some cells/debris	25	20 (80)	70
Many immotile sluggish/erratic	20	12 (60)	50
Massive clumping	10	5 (50)	45
Tail agglutination many immotile	12	5 (41)	41
Massive cells/debris	7	2 (30)	30
Results with various groups of patients			
Tubal	95	87 (92)	85
Oligospermic*	31	23 (74)	65
'Idiopathic'	10	9 (90)	80

* Fertilization rates depend on the presence of agglutination, inflammatory cells, etc. in semen.

advance the timing of laparoscopy because the beginning of the LH surge indicates oocyte recovery at some impossibly early hour in the morning. In such circumstances, the oocytes are collected in late evening, and are matured overnight in a mixture of follicular fluid and culture medium. The procedure was introduced some years ago when delays arose during the collection of sperm by individual men. Even when insemination is delayed, many oocytes retain an excellent morphology *in vitro*. They can be fertilized, will cleave normally, and produce pregnancies. Much more information is needed on the degree of success with such treatments, in comparison with the use of oocytes which are fully mature when aspirated from their follicle and inseminated immediately and such data will accumulate over the coming years. One clinic has reported that two oocytes matured *in vitro* for longer periods developed into live births[9]. Obviously, the successful maturation of oocytes *in vitro* would relieve many of the pressures on the timing of operations for oocyte collection. If, for example, oocytes could be collected at 15–20 h after the LH surge, matured *in vitro*, fertilized and developed into embryos, and then implanted at rates similar to those collected later, then the clinical convenience could be considerable.

There is also much evidence to show that fertilization can be delayed for some time, without precluding the chance of pregnancy. In two of our patients at least, fertilization was delayed by many hours – perhaps up to 20 hours – after the oocytes were aspirated from their follicles (Table 3). Yet the embryos developed *in vitro*, and some appeared to cleave more quicly and normally as if they were 'catching up' on the developmental programme, and two healthy children were born. We would not counsel that insemination is routinely delayed after oocyte aspiration, but it is comforting to know that delays in the collection of spermatozoa, or some other unforeseen difficulty leading to a delayed insemination, do not necessarily prevent a successful outcome to the treatment. This evidence is also fascinating in showing that delayed fertilization can lead to normal diploid development in man, because it is associated with polyspermy and digyny in animal eggs[10]. Perhaps the human oocyte can retain its block to polyspermy for long periods under the conditions used for culture, and it is even possible that their storage in a mixture of culture media and follicular fluid is preferable to conditions in the oviduct, which may predispose to polyspermy.

Table 3 Timing of embryonic development *in vitro* in two cases of prolonged delay in insemination [10]

Hours after beginning of LH surge	*Hours after oocyte recovery*	*Stage of development*	*Development of freshly inseminated embryos*[8]
		Patient 1	
34	8	Insemination	–
56	30	1-cell (no pronuclei)	
59	33	1-cell (additional sperm added)	
84	58	? syngamy	4-cell
87	61	3-cell	
108	81	6-cell	8/16-cell
110	83	6-cell embryo replaced into mother	
		Patient 2	
42	19	Insemination	
58	35	1-cell	
83	60	4-cell	4-cell
92	69	8-cell	4-cell
94	71	8-cell embryo replaced into mother	

The greatest problem concerning IVF still remains the induction of implantation, a difficulty that has faced us since 1970. The rates of implantation are still depressingly low in some clinics, and it is obvious that standards of quality control all stages of follicular growth, ovulation, laparoscopy, fertilization and cleavage *in vitro* and embryo replacement are essential if satisfactory success is to be obtained through IVF. The first problem to solve undoubtedly concerns the method of replacement of embryos. We have developed a catheter, called the Wallace catheter, which is simple, non-toxic, and very easy to use. With skill, it can be passed simply and easily through the cervical canal, adapting its shape to the canal as it moves forward. It can be given some support if needed by a stiffer movable outer catheter. The whole procedure of replacing embryos, from the loading of embryos into the catheter to the final check to make sure the embryos have left it, can take less than 1 minute. The procedure is non-traumatic, performed without anaesthesia, but very skilful, and the last factor is perhaps instrumental in gaining high rates of success. In our work in Bourn Hall, success rates have exceeded 30% in 1983 (Table 4), which is a wonderful tribute to the skill of the people working in embryo growth and replacement.

Table 4 Analysis of the incidence of pregnancy and abortion following embryo replacement[7]

Date	*No. of patients replaced*	*No. (%) with clinical pregnancies*‡	*Incidence of abortion (%)*
Oct '80– 5 Mar '82	515*	85 (16.5)	24 (28.2)
6 Mar '82–18 Sept '82	316†	52 (16.5)	18 (34.6)
19 Sept '82–31 Dec '82	162	38 (23.5)	10 (26.3)
1 Jan '83–28 Feb '83	82	24 (29.2)	
1 Mar '83–30 Apr '83	125	36 (28.1)	

*'Biochemical' pregnancies identified in 15 of these patients.
†'Biochemical' pregnancies identified in 5 of these patients.
‡These have not been included as clinical pregnancies.

Some detailed evidence is now indicating the nature of some of the factors that may be involved in the implantation of embryos. There is no doubt that replacing two or more embryos is more successful than replacing one. Indeed, it is only this observation which has led us to abandon the natural menstrual cycle and use stimulated cycles. I would like to point out, however, that the incidence of pregnancy in our hands using the natural cycle is much higher than in other clinics using stimulated cycles and replacing two or more embryos. The rate of implantation when clomiphene is combined with an LH surge is approximately 16% with one embryo, 31% with two embryos and 38% with three, which reflects a binomial progression in the rate of implantation (Table 1). The results are obviously highly encouraging. These data were obtained until the end of 1982; recently success rates have increased even more.

A slightly lower result is obtained from our patients given clomiphene and hCG to induce ovulation (Table 1). In them, the rates of implantation were lower with one, two or three embryos, even though the same embryologists were using the same methods on both groups of patients. This observation is most interesting. Embryos arising from clomiphene/hCG might be slightly less durable than those obtained after clomiphene and an LH surge as discussed earlier. On the other hand, poorer endocrine conditions in the mother might arise after the use of hCG as compared with an LH surge, which would not be surprising to physiologists. There are, at present, no studies on the endometrium to find out if these two forms of treatment result in differing uterine responses. It is possible to develop statistical models based on our observations which explain why success with clomiphene/hCG is far less successful than with clomiphene/LH surge, especially when three or more embryos are replaced. It is, indeed, highly essential to develop such models, and to develop parameters to estimate the success of embryonic growth, maternal capacity to implant one or more embryos and individual variations in response to treatments. Success can be influenced by various factors, e.g. maternal age (Tables 5 and 6). Such knowledge would enable us to produce the most effective treatment for individual patients, which must be the primary target for all of us. At present, we would recommend clomiphene with an LH surge as preferable treatment, followed by clomiphene combined with hMG and an LH surge. This is again the reason why we believe it is essential to monitor closely the follicular phase of our patients within the Clinic, and so increase the chances of implantation.

An obvious benefit arises from the replacement of two or more embryos or the occurrence of some multiple pregnancies. We have had many twins and rare triplet pregnancies, especially with clomiphene/hCG (Table 7). How curious that the incidence of implantation is greater with clomiphene/LH, but the incidence of multiple pregnancy is greater with clomiphene/hCG. Obviously, the birth of twins is helpful to many mothers, enabling them to establish their family at one attempt, and this must be an important factor in our calculations of the success of IVF.

Table 5 Effect of age on implantation (until December 31 1982)

Age of patients	*Natural cycle*		*Clomiphene/LH surge*		*Clomiphene/hCG*	
	Total no.	*No. (%) with clinical pregnancies*	*Total no.*	*No. (%) with clinical pregnancies*	*Total no.*	*No. (%) with clinical pregnancies*
20–24	3	0	4	0	1	0
25–29	42	7 (16.7)	49	10 (20.4)	32	7 (21.9)
30–34	116	19 (16.4)	158	42 (26.6)	101	18 (17.8)
35–39	89	12 (13.5)	136	22 (23.5)	102	16 (15.7)
40+	6	0 (0)	29	1 (3.4)	14	1 (7.1)
20–39	250	38 (15.2)	347	74 (21.3)	236	41 (17.4)

Table 6 Maternal age and abortion

Age and number of embryos replaced	*All stimulated cycles*		*Natural cycle*		*Overall %*
	No. pregnant	*No. aborted*	*No. pregnant*	*No. aborted*	
25–29:					
Single	5	2	7	0	16.7
Multiple	12	3			25
30–34:					
Single	30	6	19	7	26.5
Multiple	35	11			31.4
35–39:					
Single	19	4	12	7	35.5
Multiple	22	10			45.5
40+:					
Single	2	1			50
Multiple	2	2			100

Overall data: Single replacements in stimulated cycles, 23.2%; Single replacements in natural cycle, 36.8%; Multiple replacements in stimulated cycles, 36.6%.

Table 7 Incidence of multiple pregnancy

No. of embryos replaced	*Clomiphene/LH surge*		*Clomiphene/hCG*	
	Single	*Twin*	*Single*	*Twin*
2	9	3	11	8
3		1		

Why, then, do more twins arise with clomiphene/hCG which is less successful if one embryo is replaced? Once again, it is essential to try to understand the factors involved, and to produce statistical models which enable us to predict the best interests of each patient. At present, we can explain theoretically the high incidence of twins with clomiphene/hCG, and the lower incidence of implantation with this treatment through the poorer ability of mothers to implant their embryos[11]. Clearly, studies on implantation – on its endocrinology, physiology and statistics – are now urgently needed because success rates through embryo replacement might even surpass those attained following conception *in vivo* during the natural menstrual cycle. Many commentators have predicted that the success of IVF will maximize at approximately 25% of replacements, i.e. the rate during natural conception. I have always disagreed with this pessimistic outlook on the success of IVF.

By now, more than 110 babies have been born from work in Bourn Hall, and another three from the earlier work in Oldham, and more than 300 pregnancies have been established. We believe that these figures represent approximately one-half of the world's total. None of the children has any serious physical anomaly, hence we can conclude that IVF does not appear to be associated with any teratological damage to the child. Follow-up studies on the children are needed, and are being carried out in Bourn Hall, and no overt problems have arisen with the growth of these children up to the age of 5 years. There is a slight excess of girls among the children, whereas a slight excess of boys occurs after conception *in vivo*; we have insufficient information to decide if this difference is significant.

There is no doubt now that IVF is an acceptable and desirable treatment of infertility, becoming widely practised, and simpler with increasing experience. Further increase in success rates will result in it becoming the primary treatment of female infertility and some forms of male infertility. Such indices of success imply that new clinical treatments may soon be introduced: e.g. the identification of embryos with genetic defects. Already, DNA probes are being introduced which can identify characteristics in a few cells, e.g. probes for the Y chromosome in mice[12], and other Y probes may be effective with human tissues. Identifying the sex of an embryo through the sex-determining genes on the Y chromosome would be a beginning for such a genetic programme, and would indicate its potential by showing that heterozygous (carrier) embryos can be identified. Perhaps, too, the study of embryos *in vitro* until slightly later stages of growth – now increasingly accepted by many authorities pronouncing on the ethics of IVF – would yield stem cells capable of repairing haemopoietic, neural, myocardial and other tissues in children and adults. These exciting possibilities are becoming closer as the advantages of IVF become apparent.

The introduction of IVF into clinical practice on a wide scale has also led to many fundamental studies on human reproduction. So many studies have begun or are impending: e.g. endocrinological studies on the astonishing diurnal rhythm in the timing of the LH surge and, inevitably, of ovulation in women; the close relationship between the daily LH rhythm and the daily cortisol rhythm; and the analysis of inhibin and other factors in follicular fluid. Studies on gametes include the karyotyping of human oocytes to find out the causes of chromosomal imbalance, the identification of defective spermatozoa at the ultrastructural level, and the use of probes to find out deficient elemental components. Embryonic studies include the factors leading to polyspermy in eggs, the conditions necessary for the growth of embryos to blastocysts and their hatching from the zona pellucida and the differentiation of embryonic stem cells. These are opportunities offering the widest scope for research. I have commented on these elsewhere, and would merely like to draw attention to them here.

IVF has now come of age. It has proved successful, acceptable, simple, and capable of being adapted on a wide scale. It will be fascinating to discuss developments at the next meeting of the International Federation of Fertility Societies, and we can predict that considerable progress will be made on many areas of medical and scientific research by then.

Acknowledgements

I wish to thank my colleagues at Bourn Hall for their sustained support during this work, especially Patrick Steptoe, Simon Fishel, Jean Purdy and John Webster.

References

1. Steptoe, P.C. and Edwards, R.G. (1970). *Lancet*, **1**, 683
2. Lenz, S. and Lauritsen, J.G. (1982). *Fertil. Steril.*, **38**, 673
3. Wikland, M., Nilsson, L., Hansson, R., Hamberger, L. and Janson, P.O. (1983). *Fertil. Steril.*, **39**, 602
4. Feichtinger, W. and Kemeter, P. (1983). Presented at the *Conference on the In Vitro Fertilization of the Human Egg*, Vienna
5. Edwards, R.G. and Steptoe, P.C. (1975). *J. Reprod. Fertil.*, Suppl. **22**, 121
6. Fowler, R.E., Edwards, R.G., Walters, D.E., Chan, S.T.H. and Steptoe, P.C. (1978). *J. Endocrinol.*, **77**, 161
7. Edwards, R.G. and Steptoe, P.C. (1984). (In press)
8. Edwards, R.G., Purdy, J.M., Steptoe, P.C. and Walters, D.E. (1981). *Am. J. Obstet. Gynecol.*, **141**, 408
9. Veeck, L.L., Wortham, J.W.E., Witmyer, J., *et al.* (1983). *Fertil. Steril.*, **39**, 594
10. Fishel, S.B., Edwards, R.G. and Purdy, J.M. (1984). (In preparation)
11. Austin, C.R. (1961). *The Mammalian Egg*. (Oxford: Blackwell Scientific Publications)
12. Singh, L. and Jones, K.W. (1982). *Cell*, **28**, 205

Part IV

Section 2 Cryopreservation in Animals

31
Successful cryopreservation of eight-cell rabbit embryos using an 'open freezing system'

S. AL-HASANI, S. TROTNOW, M. BARTHEL and J. MÜLLER

Whittingham *et al.*[1,17] were the first to obtain viable offspring from mice embryos stored at −196°C transferred to recipients. Only in this species were the results of frozen–thawed embryos comparable with those obtained with unfrozen embryos. In certain other mammalian species, the survival rate of frozen embryos is not optimal when compared with that of unfrozen embryos, particularly after transfer to recipient animals. Viability of frozen embryos after transfer is very low in rabbits. Only 7–15% of the 8-cell embryos showed normal development after transfer to foster mothers[1–9,15,16]. Better results were only exceptionally obtained with morulae stage[4,10]. The benefit of an 'open freezing system' upon the developmental capacity of frozen–thawed mice and rabbit embryos was published previously[11,12]. Why rabbit eight-cell embryos stored at −196°C have low viability remains unclear.

In this study we have examined the effect of different synchronization between donor and recipient upon the transfer results of eight-cell rabbit embryos stored at −196°C[13,14].

Rabbit eight-cell embryos were collected from superovulated animals 36–40 h after the instrumental insemination and LH injection. 1.5 mol of DMSO was used as a cryoprotective agent. Two different freezing programmes (long and rapid) were used to freeze the eight-cell embryos to −196°C. These embryos were stored in liquid nitrogen for 10–60 days.

After thawing by using different warming temperatures (in air or water bath) these embryos were either cultured for 4 h before they were transferred to foster mothers or cultured in Ham's F10 for 4–5 days until they reached the blastocyst stage.

Table 1 shows the developmental capacity of frozen–thawed embryos which were slowly frozen to −70°C and cultured for further 4–5 days.

Table 1 *In vitro* development of eight-cell rabbit embryos frozen to −196 °C in 1.5 mol l^{-1} DMSO at a cooling rate of 0.5 °C min^{-1} to −70 °C and warmed at 0 °C and room temperature

Rate of warming (°C min^{-1})	*No. of embryos frozen/no. of embryos found after thawing*	*No. (%) intact embryos after thawing*	*No. (%) blastocysts 4–5 days after culture*
50	60 / 58	31 (53.4)	36 (62.0)
25	66 / 63	52 (82.5)	56 (88.8)

By using the slow-freezing programme the developmental capacity of frozen eight-cell embryos was better according to the number of intact and developed blastocyst after thawing, as shown in Table 1. The thawing rate of 25°C min^{-1} in room temperature was superior to thawing in an ice bath. 56 (88.8%) embryos reached the blastocyst stage.

Using the rapid-freezing programme the blastocyst stage was reduced to 56.8%, as shown in Table 2.

Table 2 *In vitro* development of eight-cell rabbit embryos frozen to −196 °C in 1.5 mol l^{-1} DMSO at a cooling rate of 0.3 °C min^{-1} to −30 °C and warmed in 5 °C and 15 °C water bath

Rate of warming (°C min^{-1})	*No. of embryos frozen/no. of embryos found after thawing*	*No. (%) intact embryos after thawing*	*No. (%) blastocysts 4–5 days after culture*
200	62 / 59	36 (61.0)	19 (32.2)
400	89 / 88	61 (69.3)	30 (56.8)

Of 151 embryos, 147 were found after thawing. Sixty-two embryos were thawed in a 5°C water bath and 36 embryos were seen to be intact as an eight-cell stage. From these, 19 (32.2%) embryos reached blastocyst stage after 4–5 days culture. Sixty-one (69.3%) embryos were intact when 89 embryos were thawed in a 15°C water bath and 50 (56.8%) embryos developed to blastocyst. These results indicate that

Table 3 Development of rabbit embryos frozen to −196 °C after thawing and after transfer to different asynchronous foster mothers

Recipient no.	*Length of the luteal phase of cycle (L)*	*No. of embryos transferred*	*No. (%) of implantations at day 15*	*No. of fetuses*	*No. of resorptions*	*No. of live offspring*
4	22	44	8 (18.0)	5	3	5
5	16	55	29 (53.0)	28	1	27
7	10	51	23 (45.0)	20	3	20

thawing in a 15°C water bath is superior to thawing at 5°C in respect to the developmental capacity of the embryos.

Table 3 shows the results of frozen embryos transferred to different asynchronous foster mothers. The implantation rate was high (53.0%), when the recipient were injected with LH 16 h before transfer of frozen–thawed embryos. A good result (45.0%) was achieved with recipient injected 10 h before doing embryo transfer. A total of 52 live offspring were born 28–30 days after embryo transfer.

In the literature, eight-cell embryos were frozen only by using a slow freezing programme and the developmental capacity *in vitro* was between 40 and 77%[1,3,7,10]. Our results with the slow-freezing programme were optimal but using the rapid-freezing programme the developmental capacity was similar to the results achieved by other investigators.

Our observation shows that eight-cell embryos developed slowly after thawing until they reached the 16-cell stage and after the development went on normally until the blastocyst stage. Because of this different asynchronous recipients were used. By using −6 h asynchronous recipients the *in vivo* development was 9.2% but the best implantation rate of 53% was achieved by using −24 h asynchronous recipients. When these results are compared with the implantation rate given in the literature, this is the first report with a high rate of implantation from frozen–thawed rabbit eight-cell stage. A higher implantation rate can be achieved by using only good intact embryos after thawing to reach the implantation rate of frozen–thawed morula stage as was given in the literature. All the born offsprings were fertile until the third generation.

References

1. Whittingham, D.G. and Adams, C.E. (1976). Low temperature preservation of rabbit embryos. *J. Reprod. Fertil.*, **47**, 269
2. Bank, H. and Maurer, R.R. (1973). Survival of frozen rabbit embryos. *Cryobiology*, **10**, 508 (Abstract)
3. Landa, V. (1981). Factors influencing the results of transfers of rabbit embryos stored at −196°C. *Fal. Biol. Praha*, **27**, 265

4. Maurer, R.R. and Haseman, K. (1976). Freezing morula stage rabbit embryos. *Biol. Reprod.*, **14**, 256
5. Ogawa, S. and Tomoda, S. (1976). Survival of 16-celled and morula stage rabbit embryos frozen to −196°C. *Exp. Anim. (Tokyo)*, **25**, 273
6. Parvex, R., Renard, J.P. and Ozil, J.R. (1980). Viability of rabbit embryos after freezing in liquid nitrogen. Presented at the *Ninth International Congress of Animal Reproduction and Artificial Insemination*. 3rd Symposia, 16–20 June 1980, Spain. p. 464
7. Schneider, U., Hahn, J. and Sulzer, H. (1974). Erste Ergebnisse der Tiefgefrierkonservierung von Mäuse- und Kanincheneizellen. *Dtsch. Tierärztl. Wochenschr.*, **81**, 445–76
8. Schneider, U., Görding, G., Al-Hasani, S. and Hahn, J. (1981). Survival of frozen rabbit blastocysts after rapid thawing. III. Presented at the *World Congress of Human Reproduction*, 1981, Berlin 22–26 March
9. Tsunoda, Y., Soma, T. and Sugic, T. (1981). The survival of rabbit morulae preserved in liquid nitrogen after rapid thawing. *Jpn. J. Anim. Reprod.*, **27**, 157–60
10. Bank, H. and Maurer, R.R. (1974). Survival of frozen rabbit embryos. *Exp. Cell Res.*, **89**, 188
11. Al-Hasani, S., Trotnow, S. and Köhnlein, M. (1983). Kryokonservierung von Mäuseembryonen nach dem Zwei-Stufen-Verfahren im automatisierten 'offenen System'. *Zuchthygiene*, **18**, 7–13
12. Al-Hasani, S., Trotnow, S. and Barthel, M. (1982). Kryokonservierung von Kaninchenembryonen des Acht-Zell-Stadiums im automatisierten 'Offenem System'. *Geburtshilfe und Frauenheilkunde*, **12**, 847–908
13. Al-Hasani, S. (1980). *In vitro Befruchtungsversuche mit praeovulatorischen Kanincheneizellen*. Hannover, Tierärztliche Hochschule, Dissertation
14. Al-Hasani, S., Trotnow, S. and Sadtler, Ch. (1982). Die Bedeutung der Synchronität für den Embryotransfer nach *in vitro*-Fertilisation von praeovulatorischen Kaninchenoozyten. VII. Veterinär-Humanmedizinische Gemeinschaftstagung, Giessn, 18–20, February
15. Tsunoda, Y. and Sugic, T. (1977). Effect of the freezing medium on the survival of rabbit eggs after deep freezing. *J. Reprod. Fertil.*, **50**, 123–24
16. Whittingham, D.G. and Adams, C.E. (1974). Low temperature preservation of rabbit embryos. *Cryobiology*, **11**, 560–1 (Abstract)
17. Whittingham, D.G., Leibo, S.P. and Mazur, P. (1972). Survival of mouse embryos frozen to −196°C and −296°C. *Science*, **178**, 411–14

Part V

Ethical and Legal Aspects

32
In vitro fertilization and embryo transfer: Jewish ethical and legal aspects

J.G. SCHENKER

The practice of *in vitro* fertilization and embryo transfer (IVF and ET) and especially its future potential applications creates ethical, legal and religious problems which have special implications with regard to implementation of this procedure in different societies, especially in Israel, a country where jurisdiction in matters of personal status is governed by the religious, as well as the civil authorities.

At present IVF and ET technique is acceptable in most countries but restricted only to lawfully married couples where the clinical aim is to assist them in bearing children of their own. The technique provides the possibility of oocyte donations, sperm donations, embryo donations and the use of surrogate mothers. Some opponents of IVF and ET have expressed concern regarding potential 'horrors' of future applications of this technique, such as eugenic control of birth, embryo manipulation, splitting, genetic engineering, cloning and human–animal hybrids.

Science and technology in the field of human reproduction present new and religious questions which do not always have immediate answers.

The Jewish faith is greatly concerned with the problem of reproduction. Therefore, the various aspects of the 'test-tube baby' are of considerable interest in the rabbinical literature (Response). The basic assumption in order for IVF and ET to be considered in the rabbinical literature at all, is for the oocyte and the sperm to originate from the wife and husband, respectively. The attitude favoured by the Jewish religious authorities of IVF and ET may be based on the biblical commandment: 'Be fertile and multiply. Fill the earth and master it' (Genesis 1:28).

What are some of the delineating factors which would nevertheless withhold Jewish law from preceding with IVF and ET? Some of the rabbis take a strict position and suggest that the legal and biological ties are severed with the removal of the egg. Since the host environment is sustained by medical intervention using different culture media, this may change the biological and legal status of the child. From the Jewish religious point of view, the Chief Rabbis of Israel, one of the Ashkenazi sector (European origin) and one of the Sepharadim sector (Oriental origin), support IVF and ET procedures. Jews living outside Israel are generally subjected to the laws of the country in which they live, except in cases where they wish or are required to obey the Jewish traditional personal status regulations. In such cases, the rules applicable in the State of Israel will also be applied by local rabbinical authorities, when such exist and are recognized.

Jewish law places limits on semen collection, management of menstrual problems, homologous and heterologous insemination.
These factors are considered when IVF and ET are undertaken.

The collection of semen according to the Halach (Jewish Law) may present problems, because of the prohibition of masturbation and 'seed wasting'. Masturbation is strictly condemned by the rabbinical sources. 'Thou should not commit adultery, neither by hand, nor by foot.' Coitus interruptus or withdrawal, and the use of the condom are generally prohibited on the basis of the biblical injunction against 'spilling of the seed needlessly.' In IVF technique there is a possibility of seed wastage of sperm or oocyte, which according to the Jewish religion is forbidden.

In Israel special juristic problems have arisen due to the powers vested in rabbinical courts covering matters of personal status. Although general laws in Israel are secular ones legislated by the Knesset (Israel Parliament), matters concerning marriage, divorce, paternity, legitimacy and bastardy are adjudicated according to Jewish law as determined by the rabbinical courts, which follow the Orthodox interpretation of Halacha (Jewish law). Since the rabbinical courts in Israel must recognize the legitimacy of a child's birth, the legal status of a child born through the IVF and ET procedure must be determined by them. At present there have been five Jewish children born as a result of this procedure in Israel.

SPERM DONATION IN IVF PROGRAMME

Among the religious, ethical and legal problems facing us, one concerns the donation of spermatozoa to the IVF programme for women with blocked oviducts who do not have a fertile husband.

The procedure of AID is highly controversial in the Jewish religion. Some rabbis permit AID in unusual circumstances, by suggesting a non-Jewish donor, thereby resolving the possibility of incest. It should be mentioned that the practice of AID is acceptable by part of the Jewish population in Israel according to special regulations of the Ministry of Health, while the use of donor sperm is not allowed for extracorporeal fertilization in cases of infertility due to both female and male factors.

OOCYTE DONATION

Medically oocyte donation may be required in cases of infertile women when the ovaries are covered by severe adhesions or by intestines which preclude oocyte aspiration. Oocyte donation options are open to women who are known to be carriers of a gene for serious X-linked disorders and autosomal conditions on the mother's side.

In oocyte donation it is difficult to see any ethical prohibitions in those countries where artificial insemination by a donor sperm has been accepted. If AID is acceptable an oocyte donation should be acceptable too. In Israel, according to the regulations of the Ministry of Health, it is forbidden.

EMBRYO DONATION

Medical indication for embryo donation may be applied to the couple when the reason for infertility is due to both the male and female factors. The technique may be utilized in cases of habitual abortions due to genetic abnormalities and inherited diseases, which may prevent normal child development. Embryo donation can be achieved when the ovulatory cycles of the donor and the recipient are synchronized by induction of ovulation, or by storage of the embryo. In case of embryo donation, from the legal point, a prenatal adoption can be applied. According to the regulations of the Ministry of Health in Israel, it is forbidden.

FREEZING OF EMBRYO

The controversy we foresee in the freezing of an embryo of a married couple which would be stored for several years is if a younger embryo resulting from a later ovulation and fertilization is born first. This situation may raise a juristic problem, especially in Judaic law, regarding the rights of the 'first born' concerning property inheritance and title inheritance. According to Judaic law, the moment of birth is paramount:

'Jacob by deception obtained the rights of the elder' (the first born) (Genesis 25:29).

SURROGATE MOTHER

In cases of infertility due to uterine factors when the woman is unable to carry the embryo, treatment might be indicated in the following situations:

(1) Malformations of Müllerian duct.
(2) Tubercular endometritis.
(3) Severe intrauterine adhesions (Asherman's syndrome).
(4) Uterine leiomyoma.
(5) Removal of the uterus as a result of obstetric conditions.
(6) Medical conditions that would prohibit normal pregnancy and delivery.

The practice of 'surrogate mothers' may appear attractive to women who consider pregnancy to be inconvenient to them or could interfere with their careers.

Would the law recognize the biological origin of the child, or consider only the circumstances surrounding the child's birth in deciding to which woman the baby belongs? In countries where the State Law applies in matters of personal status, the relationship of the child and the parent is established by the fact of birth. Therefore, the woman who carried the child is the lawful mother, not the genetic parents who have to adopt the child after birth. A pre-birth contract between the genetic parents and the foster mother concerning the adoption of the child must be signed. According to the Judaic law, the religion of the surrogate mother can cause further juristic and religious difficulties. In the case of a non-Jewish foster mother, the question of the religion of the infant arises even though the donors of the oocyte and sperm are Jews. Judaic law states that the religion of the child is that of his mother, i.e. it is she who gives birth, irrespective of the religion of the father or indeed of the oocyte donor.

Most of the authorities in the field of IVF and ET declare that embryo transfer between women should not be encouraged – in spite of its medical indications – for treatment of infertility due to the uterine factor, until more can be deduced about the legal and psychological relationship between the genetic parents, the 'nurse mother' and the child.

SPARE EMBRYO

According to the regulations of the Ministry of Health in Israel, IVF of the human oocyte can be performed only when the conditions for embryo transfer exist and there is a real intention of transfer. Experiments on human oocytes and embryos are to be forbidden. Therefore, when we obtain four or five embryos, we must transfer them into the uterus of the natural mother.

EXPERIMENTAL CLINICAL AND LABORATORY RESEARCH

The possibility of culturing human embryos *in vitro* beyond the blastocyst state raises ethical and legal issues concerning embryo and fetal experimentation, which may lead to clinical applications:

(1) Sex typing.
(2) Prevention of inherited disease.
(3) Embryonic tissue for grafts.

As a result of the ongoing research in the field of IVF and ET, adverse effects may occur:

(1) Interspecies fertilization, human–animal hybrid.
(2) Application of the sophisticated techniques of embryo manipulation may lead to cloning of human beings.
(3) Possibility of prolonged extracorporeal gestation and ectogenesis of human embryos and fetuses.

The adverse effects of embryo manipulation and prolonged extracorporeal gestation are considered to be unethical procedures and should not be applied to human embryos.

Therefore, each society will need to determine its own standards in the practice of IVF, and new changes in clinical applications of IVF and ET as a result of ongoing developments should be introduced in accordance with social, cultural, religious and the legal regulations adopted in each country.

Bibliography

Schenker, J.G. (1983). *In vitro* fertilization on embryo transfer. *Isr. J. Med. Sci.*, **19**, 218

Schenker, J.G. (1984). Future application of IVF and ET. Jewish ethical and legal aspects. (In press)

Part VI

Early Pregnancy in Animals and Humans

Part VI

Section 1
Early Diagnosis

33
Use of a monoclonal anti-T-cell antibody in the rosette inhibition test for detecting early pregnancy factor activity

H.-R. TINNEBERG, R.P. STAVES and L. METTLER

Early pregnancy factor (EPF) is the earliest pregnancy associated factor detectable in humans[1]. In our examinations of serum collected from women artificially inseminated, EPF activity was evident with the rosette inhibition test (RIT) just 2 days after insemination (unpublished data.

Since 1974, when Morton *et al.* first described EPF to be a pregnancy associated protein in mice, it has been detected in the wallaby, rat, sheep, pig, horse, cow and in humans[2].

EPF has yet to be clearly defined or isolated; we therefore are limited at the moment to describing EPF in terms of its effect on the RIT.

The mechanisms of EPF production are under debate. Morton and others have established that in the mouse at least two components (EPF-A, produced by the oviducts, and EPF-B, produced by the corpus luteum) are present in early pregnancy sera which are required in order to elicit the expression of EPF activity in the RIT[2]. Smart *et al.*, however, detected the presence of EPF activity in human pre-implantation *in vitro* embryo cultures. Culture media in which embryos were of the 2–16 cell stage (24–74 h) had increased RIT values, therefore suggesting that in humans, an active form of EPF can be produced by the fertilized ovum alone[3].

As various research groups have failed to be able to reproduce the RIT used for the detection of EPF originally described by Morton *et al.*[4] we have primarily modified the test by incorporating the monoclonal antibody anti-human-lyt-3 (NEN) into the RIT in order to replace the need for an anti-lymphocyte serum, while different batches of ALS raised in different rabbits often have varying activities in the RIT even though the same immunization regime was applied[3].

The monoclonal antibody used is directed against the human lyt-3 antigen located on the surface of T lymphocytes. It also has the capability of recognizing the sheep red blood cell receptor essential in spontaneous rosette formation. Only 0.25 μg of monoclonal anti-lyt-3 is required for the dilution series used for the testing of ten sera at a cost of approximately one cent per test serum. Its high specificity, purity and homogeneous quality has been an important factor in making the RIT for the detection of EPF possible.

Fresh human lymphocytes are obtained following gradient centrifugation of peripheral blood which has been diluted 1:2 with physiological saline and layered over Lymphodex (Fresenius). After adjusting to a concentration of 1×10^7 cells ml^{-1} they are pre-incubated at room temperature separately with either pregnant or non-pregnant inactivated serum for a half hour while rotating on a wheel at 10 rpm. The lymphocytes are washed twice and 50 μl of the suspension per tube is added to tubes containing 100 μl of an anti-hu-lyt-3 dilution series with 20 μl of guinea-pig complement. These are then incubated for 90 min at 37°C and spun for 5 min at 1200 rpm. Then 50 μl of SRBC, adjusted to 1×10^8 cells ml^{-1} are added, the tubes spun again for 5 min at the same speed, and then resuspended on a wheel at 10 rpm for 5 min.

The rosettes are then transferred using the capillary action of short-nose pasteur pipettes to Thoma chambers and the number of rosettes per 100 lymphocytes are determined around with the region of the chamber.

The number of spontaneous rosettes formed in the controls incubated without monoclonal antibody for each serum is considered 100% and the percentage of rosettes relative to the control is calculated at each dilution of antibody. The rosette inhibition titre was that dilution of anti-hu-lyt-3 which gave 75% or less rosette formation, compared with the internal controls.

EPF activity therefore is measured on the basis of its enhancement of the ALS or monoclonal effect on spontaneous rosette formation. As schematically shown in Figure 1, when lymphocytes are pre-incubated with non-pregnant serum numerous rosettes are formed (30–35%). However, when lymphocytes are first pre-incubated with non-pregnant serum and then incubated with ALS or monoclonal antibody, a reduction in the number of spontaneous rosettes formed is evident. This effect is enhanced when lymphocytes are pre-incubated with pregnant serum so that at higher ALS or monoclonal antibody dilutions an inhibition of rosette formation still takes place.

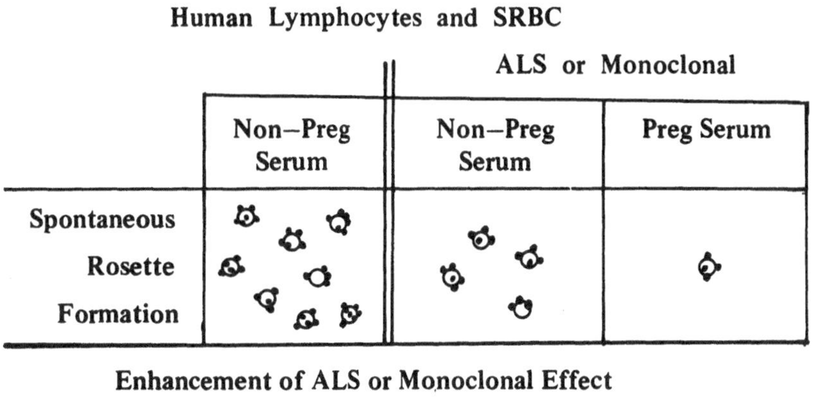

Human Lymphocytes and SRBC

		ALS or Monoclonal	
	Non–Preg Serum	**Non–Preg Serum**	**Preg Serum**
Spontaneous Rosette Formation			

Enhancement of ALS or Monoclonal Effect

Figure 1 Schematic showing the ALS or monoclonal lyt-3 sparing effect of EPF on spontaneous rosette formation following pre-incubation of lymphocytes in pregnant *vs.* non-pregnant serum

This phenomenon is shown in Figure 2. The inhibition of rosette formation by anti-hu-lyt-3 is quickly lost at low dilutions (see control). In the two cases in which lymphocytes were previously incubated with sera from women who were 7 and 10 weeks pregnant, the anti-hu-lyt-3 dilution which still caused at least 25% rosette inhibition was extrapolated to be 1:35 000 and 1:34 500 while the control RIT was only 1:9000.

The inability of many laboratories to show EPF activity in the RIT, has led to the incorporation of a monoclonal Pan-T-Cell antibody thereby modifying the original method. The increased reproducibility, subsequently obtained has reconfirmed our belief in the RIT for detecting EPF activity in early pregnancy, pregnancy following artificial insemination and in predicting disturbed pregnancies.

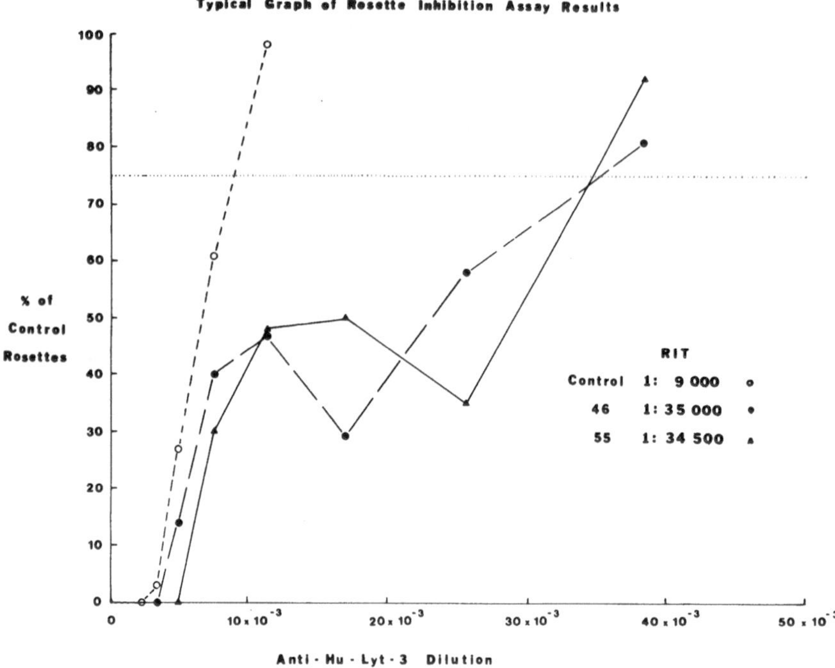

Figure 2 Rosette formation of normal lymphocytes following pre-incubation with pregnant (46, 55) and non-pregnant (control) sera showing the detection of EPF activity

References

1. Morton, H., Rolfe, B., Clunie, G.J.A., Anderson, M.J. and Morrison, J. (1977). An early pregnancy factor detected in human serum by the rosette inhibition test. *Lancet*, **1**, 394
2. Morton, H., Rolfe, B. and Cavanagh, A. (1982). Early pregnancy factor: Biology and clinical significance. In Grudzinskas, J.G., Teisner, B. and Seppälä, M. (eds.) *Pregnancy Proteins: Biology, Chemistry and Clinical Application*. pp. 391–405. (Australia: Academic Press)
3. Smart, Y.C., Roberts, T.K., Fraser, I.S., Cripps, A.W. and Clancy, R.L. (1982). Validation of the rosette inhibition test for the detection of early pregnancy in women. *Fertil. Steril.*, **37**, 779
4. Morton, H., Hegh, V. and Clunie, G.J.A. (1974). Immunosuppression detected in pregnant mice by rosette inhibition test. *Nature (Lond.)*, **249**, 459

34
A study of the accuracy of a new β hCG slide test

H. KEY and S. AVERY

A new pregnancy test, Sensislide, was introduced, with an advanced sensitivity based on a highly specific β hCG antigen. The claimed sensitivity was 0.8 IU hCG ml^{-1} and could detect a pregnancy as early as the first missed period. To determine its effectiveness, a comparison was made of the results of Sensislide with those from radioimmunoassay of β hCG.

METHOD

Radioimmunoassay of β hCG was performed on a specimen of early-morning urine and Sensislide on the same sample when a patient's period was $\geqslant$ 2 days late. Wherever possible, the number of days after ovulation on which the urine was collected was determined. Fifty-eight patients were studied.

RESULTS

In 27 patients positive Sensislides correlated with positive results found at RIA of β hCG. Twenty-three pregnancies were detected by RIA but gave a negative Sensislide result. Fifteen negative Sensislides correlated with 15 negative RIA βhCG assays. No positive pregnancies were reported as a result of Sensislide when the same urine was found to be negative using RIA.

Figure 1 indicates all the negative Sensislides with their corresponding

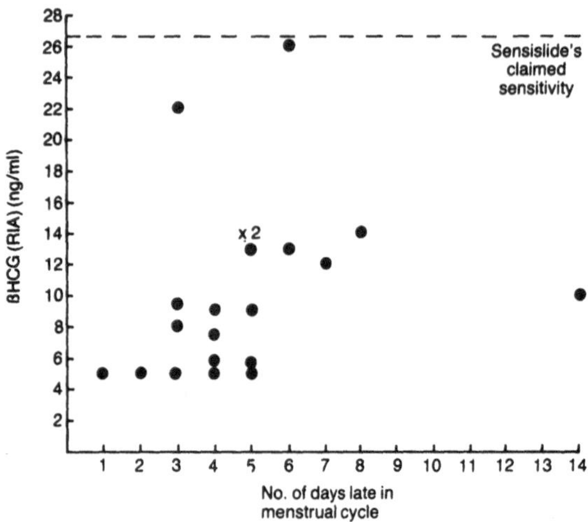

Figure 1 Negative Sensislide tests with corresponding β hCG levels as detected by radioimmunoassay

RIA values of βhCG shown against the number of days late in the menstrual cycle in which the urine was collected. All RIA values of β hCG, when there was disagreement between the two tests, fell below Sensislide's sensitivity.

However, if one looks at the relationship between the RIA values of β hCG when both tests gave a positive result and the number of days late in the menstrual cycle there is a spread of points below and above Sensislide's claimed sensitivity. Out of 27 positive correlations, 55.5% fell below this sensitivity. Hence in some patients it was confirming pregnancies below its claimed sensitivity but not in others. The earliest date at which Sensislide detected a pregnancy was 2 days late.

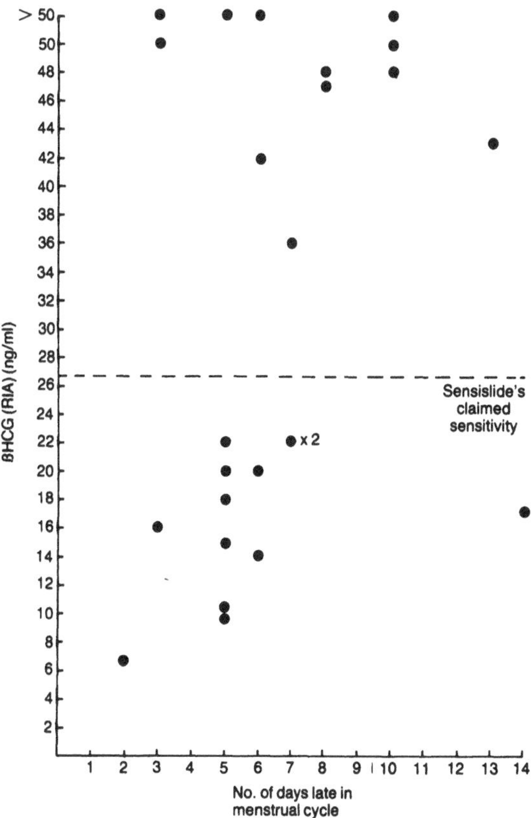

Figure 2 Positive Sensislide tests with corresponding βhCG levels as detected by radioimmunoassay

DISCUSSION

Comparing the two tests, there was a 100% correlation when the value of βhCG was above Sensislide's claimed sensitivity. Below this level there was only 39.7% correlation between the two tests. Sensislide is to be commended for detecting levels of hCG below its sensitivity but since 76% of positive results found by RIA fell below this level, it was decided to continue using this method as our main test of pregnancy.

35
Early pregnancy diagnosis in dairy cows and ewes based on milk progesterone levels

H.A. HESHMAT and A. TAHA

Progesterone levels in whole milk were determined by RIA technique in 30 native cows and ewes. A relative conformation test was performed using progesterone profile in milk for pregnancy diagnosis at 24, 40 and 44 days after insemination of cows and 18–22 days of ewes. The results revealed the following:

(1) In pregnant cows, milk progesterone profile were 5.52 ± 2.6, 6.44 ± 2.2 and 5.88 ± 1.6 mg ml^{-1} for the days 24, 40 and 44 after insemination. The accuracy of pregnancy diagnosis were 74, 85 and 92%, 24, 40 and 44 days respectively after insemination.
(2) In pregnant ewes the milk progesterone value was 4.1 ± 0.8 mg ml^{-1} in comparison with 0.6 ± 0.1 mg ml^{-1} in non-pregnant ewes; 80% of the pregnant ewes were diagnosed as pregnant.

INTRODUCTION

The discovery that the levels of progesterone in milk parallel the concentrations of this hormone in blood[1] has spurred a number of reports concerning the use of milk progesterone levels as a means for the determination of pregnancy in cows[2,3]. Encouraging results of pregnancy testing in sheep, based upon progesterone values at fixed times after breeding, have since been reported by Bassett *et al.*[4] and Robertson and Sarda[5]. The present study deals with the pregnancy test based upon RIA for milk progesterone in ewes and dairy cows.

MATERIALS AND METHODS

Thirty native cows and 30 ewes (merino) were used in this experiment. The cows and ewes were divided into two groups, pregnant and non-pregnant.

10 ml samples of whole milk were collected into plastic vials with a preservative (potassium dichromate). Samples were collected 18–22 days after mating naturally with fertile males in the case of ewes, and 24, 40 and 44 days in the case of cows progesterone assay. The progesterone content in the whole milk samples was determined by RIA after De Villa *et al.*[6].

Antiserum specificity – the cross-reactions of each antiserum to investigated hormone were also assayed.

RESULTS AND DISCUSSION

Progesterone concentration has been reported to be higher in cream than in skimmed milk[7]. The average progesterone concentration was 5.1 ng ml^{-1} in lactating non-pregnant Friesian cows, whereas in pregnant cows[1] average progesterone concentration was 19.7 ng ml^{-1}. Table 1 presents the findings regarding the progesterone concentration of whole milk at days 24, 40 and 44 days after insemination and the values obtained were 5.52 ± 2.6, 6.44 ± 2.2, 5.88 ± 1.6 ng ml^{-1}, respectively. The accuracy of pregnancy diagnosis by milk progesterone determination (Table 1) was 74, 85 and 92% at days 24, 40, 44 after insemination. The figure of 74% accuracy for positive determination at 24 days after insemination in the present study confirms the findings of Hoffman *et al.*[2] and Pennington *et al.*[3].

Table 1 Progesterone concentrations in whole milk (ng ml^{-1}) and pregnancy diagnosis in cows

Days after mating	*Progesterone*		*Correct diagnosis (%)*	
	Pregnant (n=15)	*Non-pregnant (n=15)*	*Pregnant*	*Non-pregnant*
24	5.52±2.6	0.5±0.1	74	100
40	6.44±2.2	0.2±0.05	85	100
44	5.88±1.6	0.1±0.02	92	100

The results for ewes are shown in Table 2. Milk progesterone level was higher (4.1 ± 0.8 ng ml^{-1}) in pregnant ewes than in non-pregnant ewes (0.6 ± 0.1 ng ml^{-1}) after 18–22 days from mating. On the basis of preliminary studies reported by Shemesh *et al.*[8], values above 1.5 ng progesterone (ml milk)$^{-1}$ were considered as positive for pregnancy. The results of the present study regarding the accuracy of pregnancy (Table 2) showed that 80% were diagnosed as pregnant and 94% were non-pregnant.

Table 2 Progesterone concentrations in whole milk (ng ml^{-1}) and pregnancy diagnosis in ewes 18–22 days after mating

Progesterone		*Correct diagnosis (%)*	
Pregnant (n=15)	*Non-pregnant (n=15)*	*Pregnant*	*Non-pregnant*
4.1±0.8	0.6±0.1	80	100

These results suggest that measuring progesterone levels in milk is a convenient method which substitutes for progesterone determination in blood.

References

1. Laing, J. and Heap, R. (1971). The concentration of progesterone in the milk of cows during the reproductive cycle. *Br. Vet. J.*, **127**, 19
2. Hoffman, B., Gunzler, O., Hamburger, R. and Schmidt, W. (1976). Milk progesterone as a parameter for fertility control in cattle. *Br. Vet. J.*, **132**, 469
3. Pennington, J., Spahr, S. and Lodge, J. (1976). Pregnancy diagnosis in cattle by progesterone concentration in milk. *Br. Vet. J.*, **132**, 487
4. Bassett, J., Oxborrow, T., Smith, I. and Thorburn, G. (1969). The concentration of progesterone in the peripheral plasma of pregnant ewes. *J. Endocrinol.*, **45**, 449–57
5. Robertson, H. and Sarda, I. (1971). A very pregnancy test for mammals. *J. Endocrinol.*, **49**, 407–19
6. De Villa, G., Roberts, K., Wisst, W., Milkail, G. and Flickinger, G. (1972). Progesterone determination by RIA. *J. Clin. Endocrinol. Metab.*, **35**, 438
7. Rodbard, D. and Lewald, J. (1970). Computer analysis of radioligand assay and RIA data. *Acta Endocrinol. Copenh., Suppl.*, **147**, 79
8. Shemesh, M., Ayalon, N. and Mazor, T. (1979). Early pregnancy diagnosis in ewes. *J. Reprod. Fertil.*, **56**, 301–4

Part VI

Section 2

Immunological Aspects

36
Suppressive effect of cord T lymphocytes on mixed lymphocyte reaction

F. TANAKA, Y. FUMITA, Y. MINAGAWA, C. AZUMA, F. SAJI, K. NAKAMURO and K. KURACHI

INTRODUCTION

The fetus in outbred mammalian species can survive despite disparities of participants' histocompatibility antigens. During pregnancy, maternal immune response is supposed to be suppressed by various immune suppressive mechanisms. In order to know whether cord lymphocytes can suppress the maternal immune reaction, we investigated the suppressive effect of human neonatal T lymphocytes.

MATERIALS AND METHODS

Cord blood was collected at the time of delivery. Cord lymphocytes were obtained by using a Ficoll-paque (F/H) density gradient. From the isolated cord lymphocytes, T cells were separated by using a rosette forming method at 4°C. Separated T cells were treated with mitomycin C at the concentration of 25 mg ml^{-1} for 30 min, washed, and added as regulator cells to a one-way MLR. In control study, adult T cells were treated in the same manner. One-way MLR was carried out in a flat-bottomed micro-plate with 1×10^5 responder cells, an equal number of stimulator cells, and an equal number of regulator cells in a final volume of 0.3 ml. After 5 days culture, [^{3}H]thymidine was added and DNA synthesis was assayed. All the assays were performed in triplicate and the results were expressed as the average dpm.

RESULTS AND DISCUSSION

Maternal lymphocytes response to paternal antigen was substantially suppressed by the addition of regulator cord T cells, in comparison with the response by the addition of control adult T cells. Mean percentage suppression of cord T cells on maternal lymphocyte response to paternal antigen was 36.4%. Similar suppressive effects of cord T cells were obtained in MLR response between mother and unrelated adult donors (38.9%), and donor and donor (36.3%) (Table 1). These data suggest that not only the mother's lymphocyte response but also unrelated donor's lymphocytes response in MLR were suppressed by regulator cord T cells, i.e. the suppressive effect of cord T cells is non-specific and reacts across the major histocompatibility complex barrier.

Table 1 Suppressive effect of cord T cell on various MLR

Responder	*Stimulator*	*Regulator*	*No. of cases*	*Mean suppression (%)*
Mother	Father	Cord T	5	36.4
Mother	Unrelated donor	Cord T	17	38.9
Donor	Unrelated donor	Cord T	37	36.3

In order to confirm the suppressive effect of cord T cells on MLR, various numbers of regulator cord T cells were added to the MLR consisting of 1×10^5 responder cells and 1×10^5 stimulator cells. The suppressive effect of cord T cells on MLR appeared from 3×10^4 of regulator cord T cells.

To examine the radiation sensitivity of cord T cells against suppressive effect on MLR, cord T cells were exposed to various amounts of radiation and then used as regulator cells in MLR. As a control, adult T cells were treated with the same manner. 500 and 1000 rad irradiation did not affect the suppressive effect of cord T cells and more than 2000 rad irradiation abrogated the suppressive effect (Table 2). Considering the fact that DNA synthesis of adult lymphocytes is reduced even by 250 rad irradiation, it would be reasonable to suppose that the suppressive effect of cord lymphocytes on MLR is radiation resistant.

To determine whether cord T cells exerted their suppressive effect during the early phase of MLR or late phase of MLR, time kinetics studies were carried out. Cord T cells were added at various days to MLR and its suppressive effects were examined. The strong suppression

Table 2 Suppressive effect of irradiated cord T cell on MLR

Responder	*Stimulator*	*Treatment of regulator* (rads)	*Suppression (%)*
		MMC	17
		500	29
Donor	Unrelated donor	1000	20
		2000	3
		3000	9

MMC = mitomycin C

of 27% was observed when cord T cells were added to MLR at day 0 (Figure 1). A decrease of suppressor activity was observed with cord T cells added at day 1, 2, and 3 of MLR. The results indicate that cord T cells suppress the recognition phase of MLR.

These data suggest a concept that the cord lymphocytes suppress the mother's immunological reaction against the fetal antigens.

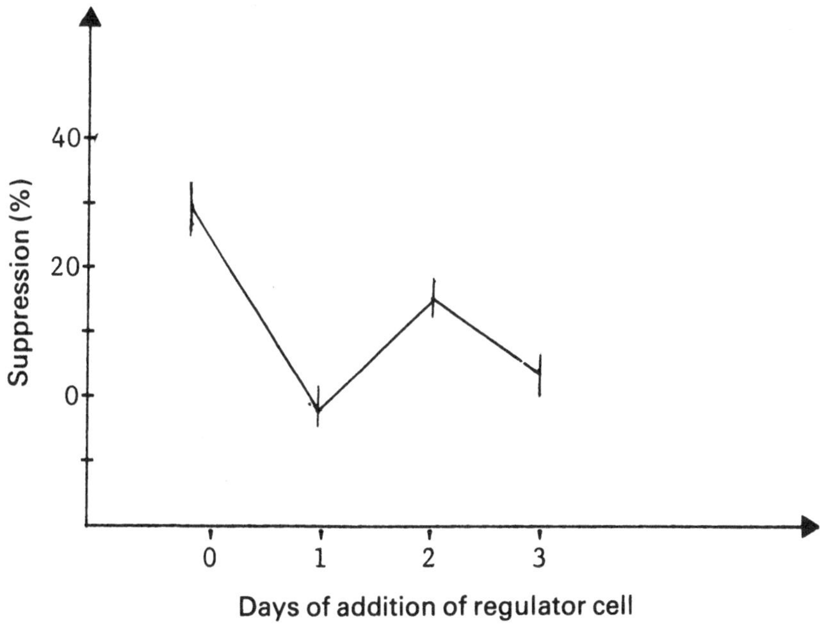

Figure 1 Kinetic study of cord T cells added at various days to MLR

37 Pregnancy associated plasma protein A: a barrier to maternal proteolytic attack

M.J. SINOSICH, D.M. SAUNDERS and J.G. GRUDZINSKAS

The placenta secretes a wide range of steroid and protein molecules into the maternal circulation. The steroids include such molecules as oestriol, and the proteins include enzymes such as heat-stable alkaline phosphatase, hormones such as placental lactogen, and a group of proteins including pregnancy associated plasma protein A (PAPP-A), which as yet have no described function[1].

Preliminary reports suggested that PAPP-A may inhibit plasmin activity and complement mediated red cell haemolysis[2] and that it may act as an immunosuppressive agent[3]. Highly purified PAPP-A was found to be a zinc carrier[4] and a non-competitive inhibitor of granulocyte elastase[5]. PAPP-A is a linear, non-competitive inhibitor of elastase. This placental glycoprotein is a specific inhibitor of granulocyte elastase as it was found to have no effect on human fibroblast collagenase, human plasmin, bovine trypsin and bovine chymotrypsin[4].

Histochemical localization of PAPP-A by the immunoperoxidase method has clearly distinguished this protein from other placental proteins such as chorionic gonadotrophin[6] and pregnancy specific β_1-glycoprotein[7]. Unlike other placental proteins PAPP-A is uniquely localized to the apical border of the synctiotrophoblast[8]. This unique distribution clearly enables PAPP-A to act locally by forming a protective sheath around the chorionic villus. Hence, the model for the action of PAPP-A as depicted in Figure 1 is proposed. The chorionic villus projecting into the intervillous blood pool is predominantly composed of trophoblastic cells and fetal blood vessels amid stromal connective tissue predominantly composed of collagen. Across the blood pool is decidual tissue interspersed with efferent and afferent maternal blood vessels. The extracellular stromal meshwork may be composed of type I, III and V collagen, while the basal membrane, in between the trophoblast cells and stromal tissue, is believed to be type IV collagen[9]. Collagen types IV and V are substrates for elastase enzymes and collagen type II is attacked by an elastase[10].

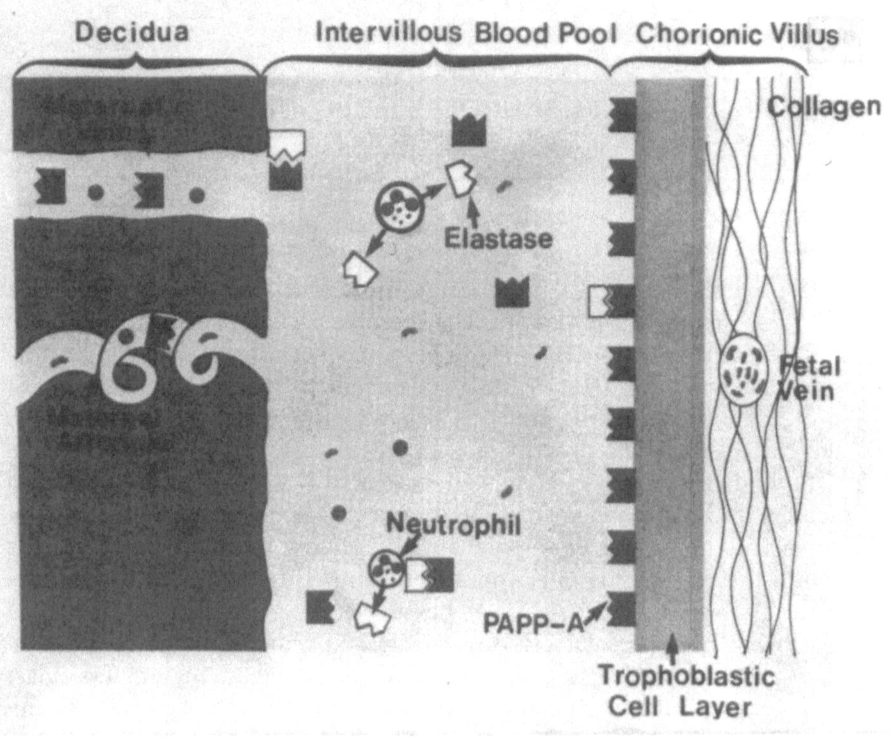

Figure 1 Model depicting a potential biological role of PAPP-A in pregnancy

Clearly the elastolytic attack directed against the chorionic villus would result in a breakdown of its structural integrity and eventual dissolution of the villus. Hence the glycoprotein barrier established at the interface between the placental cells and the maternal tissues is ideally situated to repel attack from the mother directed against the invading placenta.

PAPP-A in the maternal circulation is also functionally active as an elastase inhibitor. This protein may act peripherally to maintain proteolytic homeostasis, e.g. the presence of this protease inhibitor in the maternal circulation could also explain the remission in arthritis which occurs during pregnancy.

If this hypothesis is tenable then depressed serum PAPP-A concentration should be associated with abortion. In a recent clinical trial[11] PAPP-A was measured in the serum of 51 women who presented at hospital with clinical symptoms of threatened abortion. Those patients who aborted within 24 hours of admission were excluded from the study. Twenty of the 51 women went to term to be delivered of normal live babies, and the circulating PAPP-A levels did not differ from normal pregnancy patients. The remaining 28 women had spontaneous abortions of which 10 had positive fetal life signs as detected by ultrasonography. Only three of the 28 abortion patients had PAPP-A levels above the 10th centile, but below the median. Serial sampling on these patients showed that the rate of increase in circulating PAPP-A concentration deviated from the normal. This clearly demonstrates PAPP-A levels may determine the maintenance or loss of pregnancy.

In conclusion, appropriate levels of PAPP-A are associated with normal pregnancy outcome and we postulate that there is a critical level of PAPP-A above which the pregnancy proteolytic load is kept in check. By contrast, PAPP-A levels below this critical point are inadequate to contain the proteolytic load resulting in a placental destruction and hence pregnancy wastage. Clearly, PAPP-A is ideally situated to inhibit maternal proteolytic attack, and if the placenta acts as an allograft then PAPP-A could have a vital role in the establishment and/or maintenance of immune tolerance.

References

1. Gordon, Y.B. and Chard, T. (1979). The specific proteins of the human placenta: Some new hypotheses. In Klopper, A. and Chard, T. (eds.) *Placental Proteins*. pp. 1–21. (New York: Springer-Verlag)
2. Bischof, P. (1979). Purification and characterisation of pregnancy associated plasma protein-A (PAPP-A). *Arch. Gynaecol.*, **227**, 315
3. Bischof, P., Lauber, K., de Wurstemberger, B. and Girard, J.P. (1982). Inhibition of lymphocyte transformation of pregnancy associated plasma protein-A (PAPP-A). *J. Clin. Lab. Immunol.*, **7**, 61
4. Sinosich, M.J., Davey, M.W., Teisner, B. and Grudzinskas, J.G. (1984). Comparative studies of pregnancy associated plasma protein-A and α_2-macroglobulin using metal chelate chromatography. *Biochem. Int.* (In press)
5. Sinosich, M.J., Davey, M.W., Ghosh, P. and Grudzinskas, J.G. (1982). Specific

inhibition of human granulocyte elastase by human pregnancy associated plasma protein-A. *Biochem. Int.*, **5**, 77
6. Gaspard, U.J., Hustin, J., Reuter, A.M., Lambrotte, R. and Franchimont, P. (1980). Immunofluorescent localisation of placental lactogen, chorionic gonadotrophin and its alpha and beta subunits in organ cultures of human placenta. *Placenta*, **1**, 135
7. Horne, C.H.W., Towler, C.M., Pugh-Humpheries, R.G.P., Thompson, A.W. and Bohn, H. (1976). Pregnancy specific β_1-glycoprotein – a product of the syncytiotrophoblast. *Experientia*, **32**, 1197
8. Wahlstrom, T., Teinser, B. and Folkersen, J. (1981). Tissue localisation of pregnancy associated plasma protein-A (PAPP-A) in normal placenta. *Placenta*, **2**, 253
9. Von der Mark, K., Sasse, J., Von der Mark, H. and Kull, U. (1982). Changes in the distribution of collagen types during embryonic development. *Conn. Tiss. Res.*, **10**, 37
10. Krane, S. (1982). Collagen degradation. *Conn. Tiss. Res.*, **10**, 51
11. Westergaard, J.G., Sinosich, M.J., Bugge, M., Madsen, L.T., Teisner, B. and Grudzinskas, J.G. (1983). Pregnancy associated plasma protein-A in the prediction of early pregnancy failure. *Am. J. Obstet. Gynecol.*, **145**, 67

Part VI

Section 3
Implantation

38
Decidual cell reaction. Action of saturated and unsaturated fatty acids

P. SARTOR and G. ACKER

In several mammals including the rat, the decidual cell reaction (DCR) occurs physiologically at the time and place of ovum implantation. Its development and the appearance of a refractory state are controlled by ovarian hormones[1]. Progesterone (P) secreted during pregnancy, pseudopregnancy or injected into castrated rats is a prerequisite for DCR, but small doses of oestradiol (E_2) are needed to get a full response[1]. During the first stages of ovum implantation, prostaglandins (PGs) play an important role by increasing the endometrial vascular permeability[2]. On the other hand, recent findings by Clerc-Hofmann *et al.*[3] have demonstrated that fatty acids (FA) interact with the binding of oestradiol to its receptor. Arachidonic acid (AA) is a FA precursor of PG and in minute amounts has been described as an inducer of DCR[4]. Thus, we have tested the action of saturated (SFA) and unsaturated fatty acids (UFA), including AA, on the DCR in pseudopregnant rats.

MATERIAL AND METHODS

Female rats of the Wistar strain, housed in the laboratory and submitted to strict conditions of light and darkness, were allowed to mate with a male. The presence of the vaginal plug indicated the first day of pregnancy. Pseudopregnancy was achieved by sectioning the Fallopian tubes of both uterine horns on the 1st day. On day 5 (D5), a cotton thread, soaked in alcohol and dried, was introduced in the uterine lumen of the horn. A cotton thread soaked in pure or diluted FA and allowed to dry in the latter case was introduced into the second horn. One FA was dissolved in alcohol and allowed to dry. When FA were used undiluted 1–3 mg were introduced into the uterine lumen. The animals were killed 48 and 96 h later, the uterine horns dissected, weighed and fixed in Bouin's fluid for histological examination. The following FA purchased from Sigma were tested: palmitic acid (PA. SFA. C16:0), solubilized in alcohol, oleic acid (OA. UFA. C18:1), arachidonic acid (AA. UFA. C20:4), docosahexaenoic acid (DA. UFA. C22:6). In addition, the dose effect was studied with AA when diluted 10 and 100 times in alcohol.

RESULTS

48 h after the trauma, the growth response was similar in control and treated horns with PA. A decrease in the uterine weight of treated horns was observed with UFA (OA, AA and DA), maximal weight decrease occurring with DA (Figure 1). After 96 h, PA had little or no effect on the DCR. On the contrary, each one of the UFA was able to inhibit the DCR extensively (Figure 2). The uterine weight of treated horns was respectively 33% with OA and 26% for AA and DA of the control horn weights.

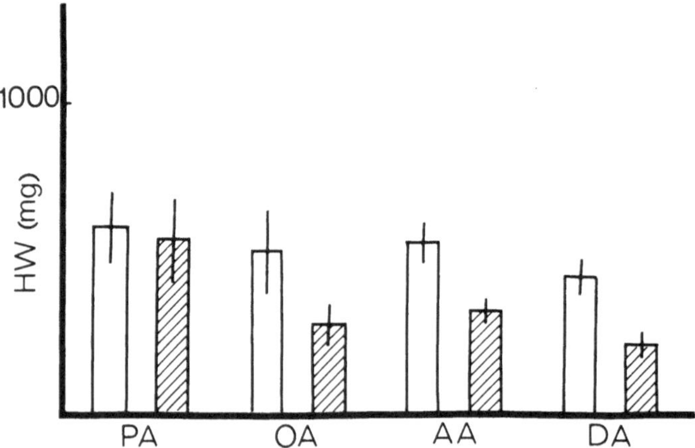

Figure 1 Ponderal evolution of the DCR in control (open bars) and treated horns (striped bars) 48 hours after trauma. Cotton threads introduced in the treated horns were soaked in palmitic acid (PA), oleic acid (OA), arachidonic acid (AA) and docosahexaenoic acid (DA). Cotton threads introduced in the control horns were soaked in alcohol and dried. HW = Mean horn weight. SE shown as vertical lines

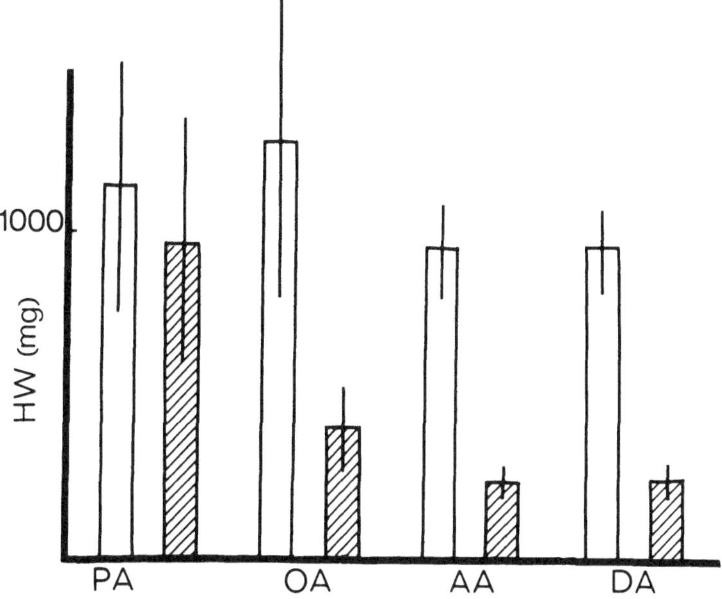

Figure 2 Ponderal evolution of the DCR in control and treated horns 96 hours after trauma. For method and abbreviations, see Figure 1

The dose–response study demonstrated that AA diluted 10-fold is not very effective in inhibiting the decidual response, and totally ineffective when diluted 100-fold (Figure 3). Histological examination of sections, 10–15 pieces for each horn, correlated well with ponderal results. With UFA, decidual nodules were occasionally seen only at the cervical or tubal end. We suppose that at these places the thread end was washed by the enteral fluid. All along the horn, we found normal stromal cells associated with inhibition of DCR.

DISCUSSION

AA is well known as a PG precursor, but OA and DA are not direct precursors. On the other hand, Clerc-Hofmann *et al.*[3] clearly demonstrated that OA, AA, DA were respectively able to interact in the binding process of E_2 with its receptor. Therefore, the action of FA on DCR development can better be correlated with their interaction in

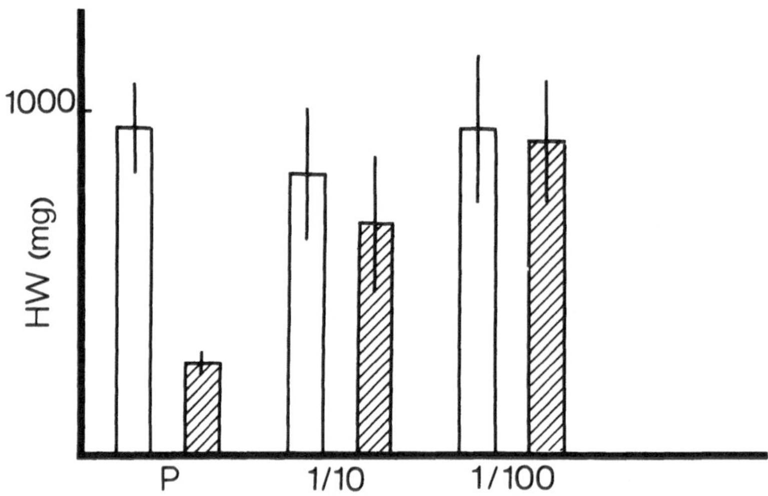

Figure 3 Dose response of the DCR. Cotton threads introduced in the treated horns were soaked in pure (P), or diluted (1/10 and 1/100) AA (in alcohol). Control horns as in Figure 1

oestradiol-receptor binding process rather than taking place in PG metabolism.

As large amounts of FA have been found in the cytosol of rat uterus[3], it is obvious that their role is to be taken into account in biological processes. In minute amounts, AA is mostly used as a PG precursor[4], but when present in excess it could also interact with oestradiol binding. We have already described a higher nuclear translocation of E_2 receptor complexes at implanted sites in the rat uterus on day 6[5]. Is the lower level of nuclear translocation found in unimplanted sites, where PG synthesis is less important, the result of such an interaction? This question is yet to be answered. Experiments are under way to verify whether the different evolution of implanted (development of the DCR) and unimplanted sites (no DCR) can be correlated with different amounts of UFA.

References

1. De Feo, V.J. (1967). Decidualization. In Wyn, R.M. (ed.) *Cellular Biology of the Uterus*. pp. 192–290. (New York: Appleton Century Crofts)
2. Kennedy, T.G. (1980). Prostaglandins in the endometrial vascular permeability changes preceeding blastocyst implantation and decidualization. In Hubinont, P.O.

(ed.) *Progress in Reproductive Biology. 7 'Blastocyst Endometrium Relationship'*. pp. 234–43. (Basel: Karger)
3. Clerc-Hofmann, F., Valette, G., Secco-Millet, C., Christeff, N., Benassayag, C. and Nunez, E.A. (1983). Inhibition de la fixation utérine des oestrogènes par les acides gras insaturés chez la rate immature. *C.R. Acad. Sci. Paris*, **296**, 53
4. Le Goascogne, C., Sananes, N. and Beaulieu, E.E. (1979). Prostaglandins and decidualization. In Crastes de Paulet, A., Thaler-Dao, M. and Dray, F. (eds.) *Prostaglandins and Reproductive Physiology*. INSERM **91**. pp. 229–42
5. Logeat, F., Sartor, P., Vu-Hai, M. and Milgrom, E. (1980). Local effect of the blastocyst on estrogen and progesterone receptors in the rat endometrium. *Science*, **207**, 1083

39
The role of vitamin E in fertility

H. KASEKI, K. SATO, Y. YOSHINO, Y. HIRAI, T. TAKESHIMA, M. TANAKA, K. SUGAWARA, T. NEMOTO and T. KASEKI

INTRODUCTION

Fetal death and resorption in rats resulting from maternal vitamin E deficiency was first observed in 1922, and extensively studied by Evans *et al.*[1]. Vitamin E is well known as an anti-sterile vitamin, but the problem is yet to be investigated as to why vitamin E prevents abortion or infertility. To clarify the problem, we determined human vitamin E concentrations of maternal plasma and normal interrupted intrauterine tissues. And we next investigated vitamin E distribution in female rats.

MATERIALS AND METHODS

We measured vitamin E levels of 39 human normal pregnant cases who were recipients of artificial interruption while in their 3rd month. Detailed gestational stages were first confirmed by gestational sac(GS) measurements[2]; that is, the longest diameter of the GS was measured by B-mode scanner before surgery. The fetal heart beat was also confirmed by B-mode scanner at this time. Maternal plasma was collected prior to surgery followed by samples of intrauterine tissues (the decidua, chorionic villi, and fetus) being collected post-operatively. They were then separated, washed with saline, and stored at −30°C. The vitamin E concentrations of the decidua, chorionic villi, fetus and maternal plasma were measured by the Two Internal Standards

Assay[3]. Since two kinds of internal standards are used, this assay method is reliable. We measured the α-tocopherol in vitamin E, because α-tocopherol is considered to have the highest biological activity naturally occurring in all the vitamin E tocopherols.

In order to investigate vitamin E distribution, four female adult rats (250–300 g) were killed and their tissues excised. Tissue vitamin E was determined by the Two Internal Standards Assay.

RESULTS AND DISCUSSIONS

Figure 1 demonstrates vitamin E distribution in the pregnant human uterus. Measured vitamin E concentrations were the highest in the decidua, and were followed by the chorionic villi and fetus. When the biological function of vitamin E is considered, a very interesting hypothesis develops. Some of the polyunsaturated fatty acids like arachidonic acid are considered to be precursors of prostaglandins[4], and they can easily alter their structures to peroxides, which in turn are considered to induce membrane disorders[1]. On the other hand, vitamin E is well known as an antioxidant that prevents polyunsaturated fatty acids from lipid peroxidation[1]. In general, prostaglandin biosynthesis is enhanced in a pregnant uterus[5], and as the illustration shows in a decidual enclosed fetochorionic unit. Therefore, a high concentration of vitamin E in the decidua prevents fetochorionic units from lipid

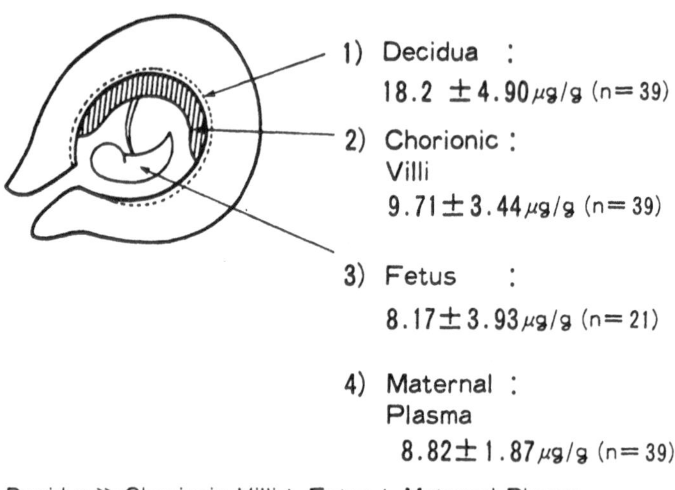

Figure 1 Vitamin E concentrations in intrauterine tissues

peroxidation in pregnant uteri, and this is considered to be the reason why vitamin E prevents abortion or infertility.

Figure 2 shows that a positive correlation was observed between fetal and chorionic villi vitamin E concentrations.

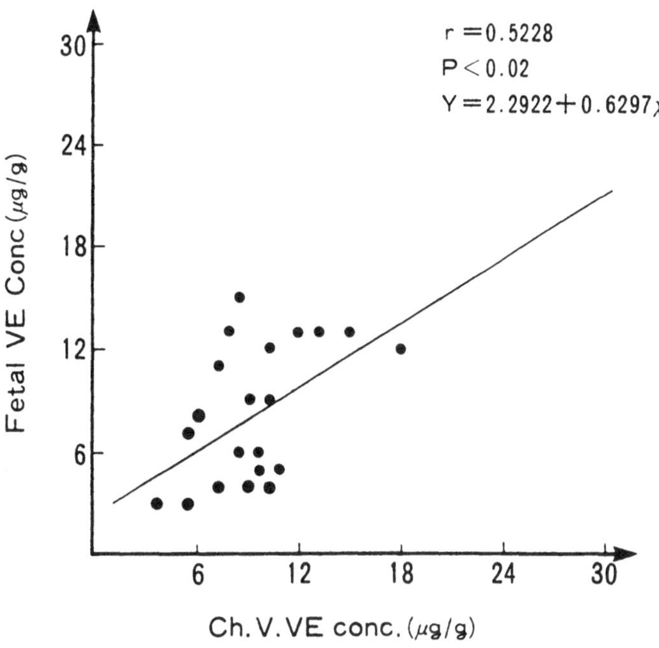

Figure 2 Correlation between fetal vitamin E (VE) and chorionic villi vitamin E (Ch. V. VE) concentrations

A negative correlation was observed between the human fetal vitamin E concentration and the longest diameter of GS (Figure 3). In general, the longest diameter of GS is considered to be indicative of fetal growth in the early stages of pregnancy[2]. This observation means that fetal vitamin E concentrations decrease as the fetus grows in the early stages of pregnancy. Conversely, very high vitamin E concentrations were expected in the blastocyst preimplantation stage.

As to vitamin E distribution in female rats, our data could not be compared with other data since no other information has been published (Table 1). Adrenal glands and ovary showed significantly high vitamin E concentrations. Since ovary and adrenal glands have a function of steroid genesis, and this result suggests that there might be

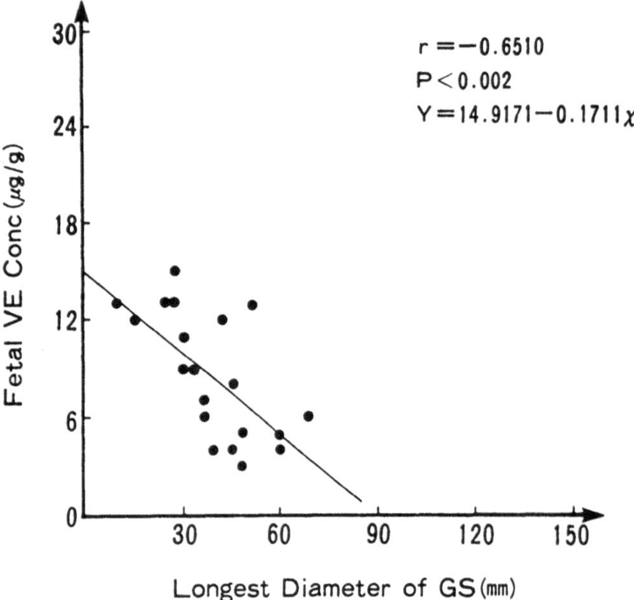

Figure 3 Correlation between fetal vitamin E (VE) and gestational sac (GS) size

some relation between vitamin E and steroid genesis. Another investigator reported that the activity of steroid genesis was decreased in vitamin-E deficient rats[6,7].

Table 1 Mean (±SD) vitamin E concentrations ($\mu g\ g^{-1}$) in four female rats

(1) Adrenal (534±78.5)	(11) Diaphragm (49.5±11.4)
(2) Ovary (497±148)	(12) Heart (48.7±10.1)
(3) Mesenteric fat (104±15.2)	(13) Liver (42.5±4.65)
(4) Renal medulla (86.2±17.0)	(14) Intestine (38.7±3.65)
(5) Bone marrow (78.7±8.36)	(15) Lung (34.3±10.4)
(6) Perirenal fat (69.8±4.63)	(16) Uterus (32.9±5.49)
(7) Skin (66.8±18.1)	(17) Renal cortex (28.9±4.09)
(8) Fallopian tube (66.3±25.7)	(18) Bone (9.96±1.42)
(9) Spleen (61.7±2.74)	(19) Eye (9.07±2.27)
(10) Muscle (61.5±4.29)	(20) Plasma (7.99±1.29)

The result of containing abundant vitamin E in ovaries and another result of decreasing fetal vitamin E in the early stages of pregnancy suggest that mammalian eggs contain abundant vitamin E which affects the maintenance of gestation. This supposition is presently under investigation by mass-chromatographic determination.

Acknowledgement

This work was partially funded by Eisai Co. Ltd.

References

1. Machlin, L.J. (ed.) (1980). *Vitamin E. A Comprehensive Treatise.* (New York: Marcel Dekker)
2. Sanders, R.C. and James, A.E. (1980). *The Principles and Practice of Ultrasonography in Obstetrics and Gynecology.* (Norwalk Connecticut: Appleton-Century-Crofts)
3. Kaseki, H., Sato, K. and Yoshino, Y. (1984). *The Quantitive Analysis of α-Tocopherol among Various Tissues in Rats. Development of The Two Internal Standards Assay.* (In preparation)
4. Samuelsson, B., Granström, G.E., Hamberg, M., Hammarström, S. and Malmsten, C. (1978). *Ann. Rev. Biochem.*, **47**, 997
5. Wallenburg, H.C.S., Zijlstra, F.J. and Vincent, J.E. (1981). *J. Dev. Physiol.*, **3**, 15
6. Barnes, M.M. and Smith, A.J. (1975). The effect of vitamin E deficiency on androgen and corticosteron synthesis. *Int. J. Vit. Nutr. Res.*, **45**, 342
7. Barnes, M.M. and Smith, A.J. (1975). The effect of vitamin E deficiency on some enzymes of steroid hormone biosynthesis. *Int. J. Vit. Nutr. Res.*, **45**, 396

Part VI

Section 4
Endocrinology. Hormone Levels in the Camel Fetus. Progesterone Therapy in Man

40
Progestin levels of the camel fetus during developmental stages

S.A.F. EL-MOUGY, F.B.S. WEHAISH and Y.M. RADWAN

INTRODUCTION

Progress in the understanding of fetal endocrinology has accelerated rapidly in the past 20 years. There is an available literature concerning fetal endocrinology in cattle[1], sheep[2] and goat[3]. Although some specific information exists on the reproductive events in camel[4–6] our present knowledge of the hormonal changes in the camel fetus is very scarce. Therefore, the present study was carried out to determine the ovarian, adrenal and plasma pregnenolone and 17α-hydroxypregnenolone levels in the camel fetus.

MATERIALS AND METHODS

Samples of blood, ovary and adrenal gland of female fetuses and samples of blood and adrenal gland of male fetuses were obtained from 150 fetuses of the pregnant one humped camel (*Camelus dromedarius*) within 1 h of their slaughter during 24 visits to Cairo abattoir between November 1982 and March 1983. Samples were grouped according to the cranio-vertebral–rump. (CVR) length of the fetus[7]. Blood samples were collected in heparinized tube and immediately centrifuged in a refrigerating centrifuge at 4000 rev/min for 30 minutes, then stored at −20°C until the day of assay. The adrenal cortex and ovary were removed immediately to be frozen at −20°C until used for hormonal assay.

Pregnenolone and 17α-hydroxypregnenolone were estimated in the plasma and tissue by RIA[8].

RESULTS

Concentration of pregnenolone and 17α-hydroxypregnenolone in the plasma and tissues are shown in Figure 1. It was found that the level of pregnenolone was higher in the ovary, plasma and slightly decreased in the adrenal of the female fetuses, together with a decrease in its level in both the plasma adrenal of the male fetuses with increase in gestational age. The level of 17α-hydroxypregnenolone was below the detectable level in the adrenal of the male and ovary of the female, while in the adrenal of the female it was slightly decreased followed by an increase at late stages of gestation.

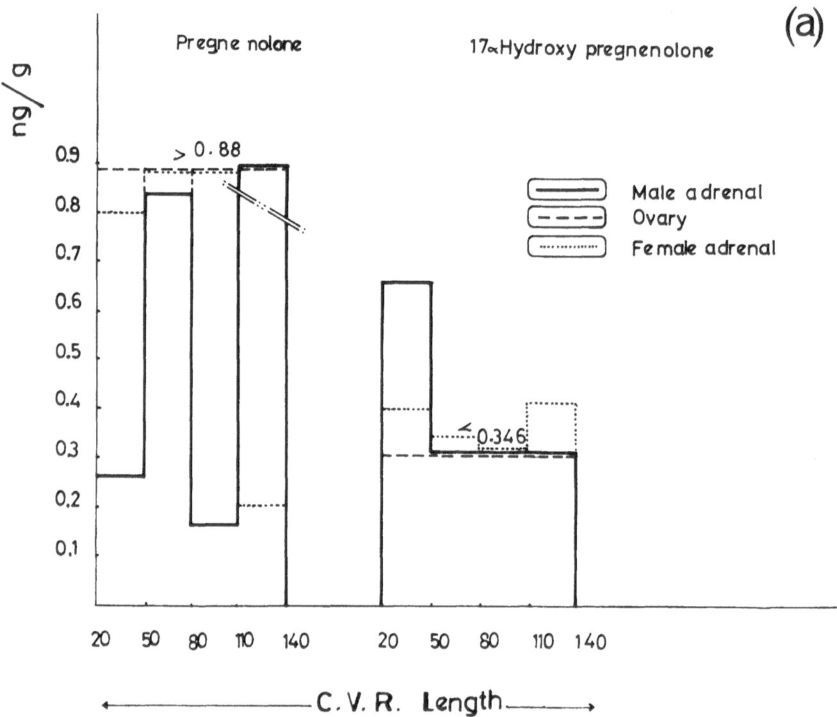

Figure 1 Concentrations of pregnenolone and 17α-hydroxypregnenolone and fetal length (*a*) in adrenal glands and ovary and (*b*) in plasma of fetuses

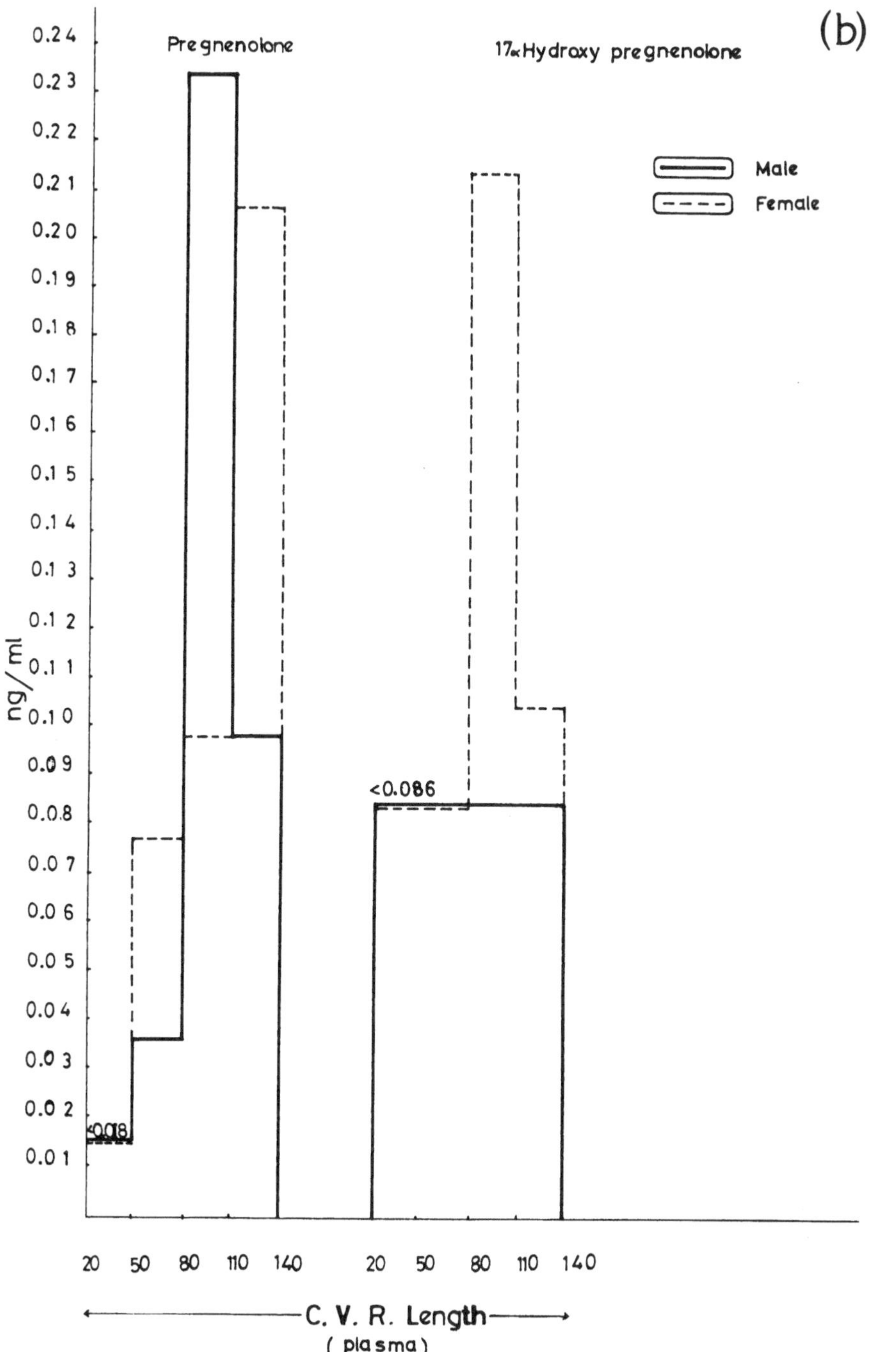
(b)
Pregnenolone
17α Hydroxy pregnenolone
Male
Female
ng/ml
0.24
0.23
0.22
0.21
0.20
0.19
0.18
0.17
0.16
0.15
0.14
0.13
0.12
0.11
0.10
0.09
0.08
0.07
0.06
0.05
0.04
0.03
0.02
0.01
<0.018
<0.086
20 50 80 110 140
20 50 80 110 140
C. V. R. Length
(plasma)

DISCUSSION

Our results show that pregnenolone slightly decreased with increase in gestational age. This confirms the well-established fact that the maternal levels of oestrogen increase and those of progesterone decline shortly before parturition in many species including sheep, goat, cow and rat. The original observations demonstrating the role of the fetal pituitary– adrenal axis in the initiation of parturition in the pregnant ewe have led to an extensive search for similar mechanisms whereby the fetus signals its readiness to enter the intrauterine environment. In sheep, increased fetal adrenal secretion of cortisol late in gestation induces the enzymes in the placenta necessary for oestrogen synthesis from progesterone[6]. Other mechanisms by which the fetus regulates progesterone production may be important in relation to the endocrine changes leading to parturition. Several investigators have suggested that regulation of progesterone synthesis may occur through pregnenolone utilization[9].

It is well established that human fetal ovarian steroidogenesis develops after 10 weeks of gestation and remains rather limited throughout fetal life. This supports our conclusion that ovarian steroidogenesis develops in camel fetus.

Therefore, it could be stated hypothetically that the source of pregnenolone in the female fetuses was from the ovary while the 17α-hydroxypregnenolone was secreted mainly from the adrenal gland[7].

References

1. Holm, L.W. (1967). Prolonged pregnancy. *Adv. Vet. Sci.*, **11**, 159–205
2. Liggins, G.C. and Kennedy, P.C. (1968). Effect of electrocoagulation of the foetal lamb hypophysis on growth and development. *J. Endocrinol.*, **40**, 333–44
3. Van Rensburg, S.J. (1971). Reproductive physiology and endocrinology of normal and habitually aborting Angora goats. *Onderst. J. Vet. Res.*, **38**, 1–26
4. Abdo, M.S., Al-Janabi, A.S. and Al-Kafawi, A.A. (1969). Studies on the ovaries of the female camel during the reproductive cycle and in conditions affected with cysts. *Cornell Vet.*, **IIX**, 418
5. Abdo, M.S. and El-Mougy, S.A. (1976). Hormonal variations in the blood of the one humped camel during the various reproductive stage. Part 2. Free estrogen content in the ovaries and blood. *J. Vet. Med. Vet. Med. Cairo Univ.*, **24**, 71
6 Ismail, A.A. (1983). *Physiological Studies on Some Reproductive States of She Camel (Camelus Dromedarius).* PhD Thesis, Veterinary Science, Faculty of Veterinary Medicine, Zagazig University, Egypt
7 Safa, O.A.F. (1962). *Prenatal Development of some Endocrine Glands. The Thyroid Gland of Camel Embryos* MSc Thesis, Faculty of Agriculture, Ein Shams University, Egypt
8 Abraham, G.E. (1977). *Handbook of Radioimmunoassay.* Vol. **5**. pp. 591–656. (California: Radioassay system laboratories)
9 Pentii, K.S. and Maria, S.F. (1981). Some new thoughts on the fetoplacental unit and parturition in primates. In Miles, J.N. and John, A.R. (eds.) *Fetal Endocrinology.* pp. 1–34. (New York: Academic Press)

41
Radioimmunoassay for oestrogens in the plasma and tissues of one-humped camel fetus

F.B.S. WEHAISH, Y.M. RADWAN and S.A.F. EL-MOUGY

INTRODUCTION

Clinical syndromes characterized by abnormal gestational lengths has provided evidence which suggests that the fetus plays a vital role in determining its own delivery. Furthermore, oestrogen formation during pregnancy depends upon a gradually increasing supply of fetal adrenal precursors as gestation advances. However, the precursors for oestro-gen biosynthesis have not been elucidated, and the situation is complicated by the extensive metabolism of steroids that occurs within the fetal vascular system[1].

Earlier observation[2] suggested that oestrogen rise before term was the result of increased fetal adrenal activity leading to increased fetoplacen-tal oestrogen biosynthesis.

Although several studies were performed on the hormonal level of animal fetuses, the camel has received very little attention; therefore, the present study was undertaken to estimate the level of total oestrogen, oestrone and oestriol in plasma and tissues of the camel fetuses during prenatal development.

MATERIALS AND METHODS

Blood, adrenal cortex and ovarian tissue samples were obtained from

150 female and male camel fetuses. The samples were grouped according to the cranio-vertebral–rump (CVR) length of the fetus. Blood samples were collected in heparinized plastic tubes and immediately centrifuged at 4°C at 4000 rpm for 30 minutes, then stored at −20°C until the day of assay.

The adrenal cortex and ovarian tissues were kept at −20°C until used for hormonal assay. Total oestrogen, oestrone and oestriol were estimated by RIA procedure similar to that adopted for human plasma[3].

RESULTS

Levels of total oestrogen, oestrone and oestriol in the plasma, adrenal cortex and ovary of the female fetuses and plasma and adrenal cortex of the male fetuses are shown in Figure 1. The levels of total oestrogen and oestrone in the adrenal tissue of the male were increased in the first two-thirds of fetal growth, then decreased in the last third, while increased levels of total oestrogen and oestrone in the ovary and adrenal of the female was detected throughout fetal development. On the other hand, the levels of oestriol were below the detectable value in both male and female fetuses.

DISCUSSION

Camel fetal steroidogenesis has not been described previously so that the comparison of the present findings can be made only with other species. Our results showed increased levels of total oestrogen and oestrone in the plasma and tissue of the camel fetuses. These results confirm the findings that the high circulating oestrogen level in the fetus may promote dehydroepiandrosterone production by the fetal adrenal glands and thus promote the secretion of the principal substrate for oestrogen production. The placenta and placental membrane acting in concert constitute the fetoplacental steroidogenic unit and produce the large amount of oestrogen characteristic of human pregnancy. Thus increased secretory activity of primate fetal adrenal glands increases the supply of oestrogen precursors to the placenta directly[4]. The fetal adrenals can maintain fetal as well as maternal plasma level of oestrogen. In human embryogenesis the differerentiation of fetal ovaries as endocrine organs capable of synthesizing steroid hormones occurs between week 8 and week 10 of gestation[5]. This evidence helped to suggest involvement of the fetus in the hormonal changes during pregnancy and parturition.

Thus the presence of oestrogen during camel fetal development could be a continuation of its role, as in other mammals, to contribute to:

(1) The hormonal control of differentiation.
(2) The implantation of blastocytes and therefore the survival of both male and female embryo.
(3) Pituitary modulation during fetal life[6].

In conclusion, we hypothesize that total oestrogen and oestrone were secreted mainly from the ovary of the female fetuses and adrenal glands of the male and female fetuses.

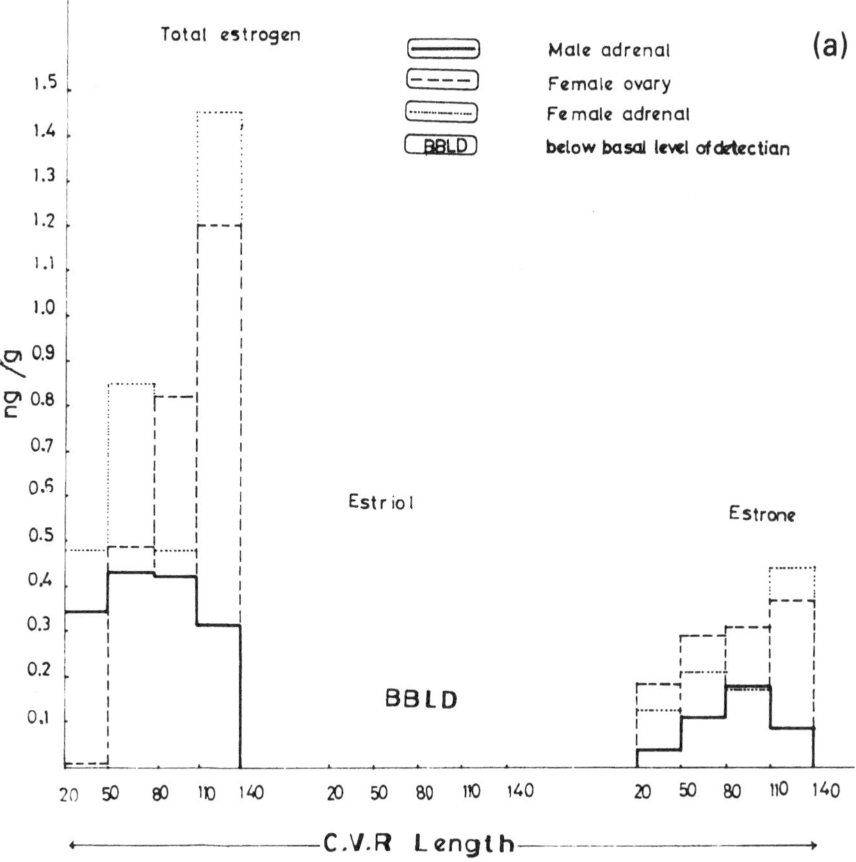

Figure 1 Oestrogen levels in (*a*) adrenal glands and ovaries and (*b*) plasma of camel fetuses

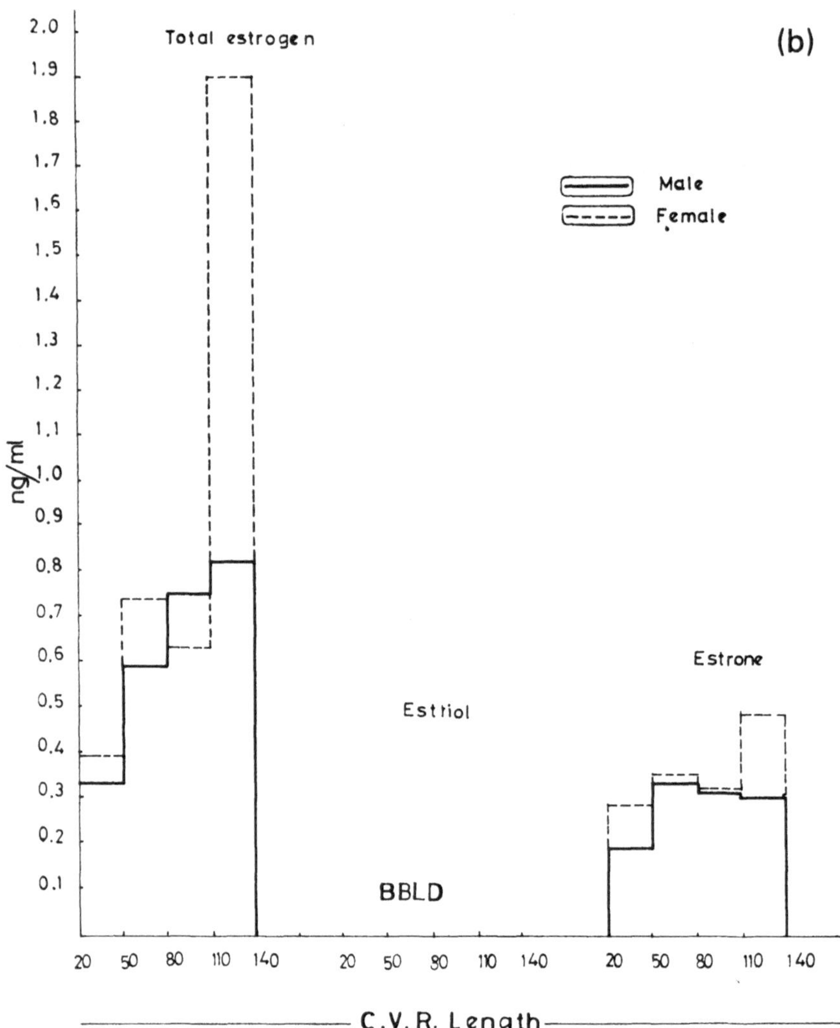

References

1. Thorburn, G.D., Challis, J.R.G. and Robinson, J.S. (1977). Endocrine control of parturition. In Wynn, R.M. (ed.) *Biology of the Uterus*. p. 666. (New York: Plenum Press)
2. Thorburn, G.D., Nicol, D.H., Bassett, J.M., Shutt, D.A. and Cox, R.I. (1972). Parturition in the goat and sheep. Changes in corticosteroids, progesterone, estrogen and prostaglandin F. *J. Reprod. Fertil.*, **16**, 61

3. Abraham, G.E. (1977). *Handbook of Radioimmunoassay*. Vol. **5**. pp. 591–656. (California: Radioassay System Laboratories)
4. Telegdy, G. and Diczfalusy, E. (1971). In James, V.H.T. and Martini, L. (eds.) *Hormonal Steroids* No. 219 in the international congress series. pp. 496–503. (Amsterdam: Excerpta Medica)
5. Pentii, K.S. and Maria, S.F. (1981). Some new thoughts on the fetoplacental unit and parturition in primates. In Miles and John, A.R. (eds.) *Fetal Endocrinology*. pp. 35–52. (New York: Academic Press)
6. Miles, J.N. and Scott, W.W. (1981). Regulation of fetoplacental steriodogenisis in rhesus macaques. In Miles, J.N. and John, A.R. (eds.) *Fetal Endocrinology*. pp. 35–357. (New York: Academic Press)

42
Plasma and tissue levels of androgens in the one-humped camel fetus

Y.M. RADWAN, F.B.S. WEHAISH and S.A.F. EL-MOUGY

INTRODUCTION

The early events in fetal life establish the biological bases of adult sexual interaction and the capacity to reproduce; thus understanding the physiological and chemical events that direct fetal differentiation and birth advances our knowledge of reproduction.

However, there is no literature on the steroid hormone levels in camel fetus. Therefore, the present work is an attempt to estimate the levels of androgens in the gonads, adrenals and plasma of the camel fetuses.

MATERIALS AND METHODS

Samples of blood, ovary and adrenals of the female fetuses and samples of blood, adrenal cortex and testes of the male fetuses were obtained from 150 female and male camel fetuses. The samples were grouped according to the cranio-vertebral–rump (CVR) length of the fetus. Blood samples were collected in heparinized plastic tubes and immediately centrifuged at 4°C at 4000 rpm for 30 minutes, then stored at −20°C until the day of assay. The adrenal cortex, ovaries and testes were kept at −20°C until used for hormonal assay.

Testosterone, 5-dehydrosterone, dehydroepiandrosterone and androstenedione were estimated by RIA procedure similar to that adopted for human plasma.

RESULTS

Levels of testosterone, dehydrotestosterone, 5-dehydroepiandrosterone and androstenedione in the plasma, adrenal and ovary of female fetuses and plasma, adrenals and testes of male fetuses are shown in Figure 1. It was found that the level of testosterone and androstenedione were markedly greater in male than in female fetuses. The level of testosterone gradually increased in male and female fetal tissue, while the level of dehydroepiandrosterone was decreased in female fetuses and gradually increased in males towards the end of pregnancy.

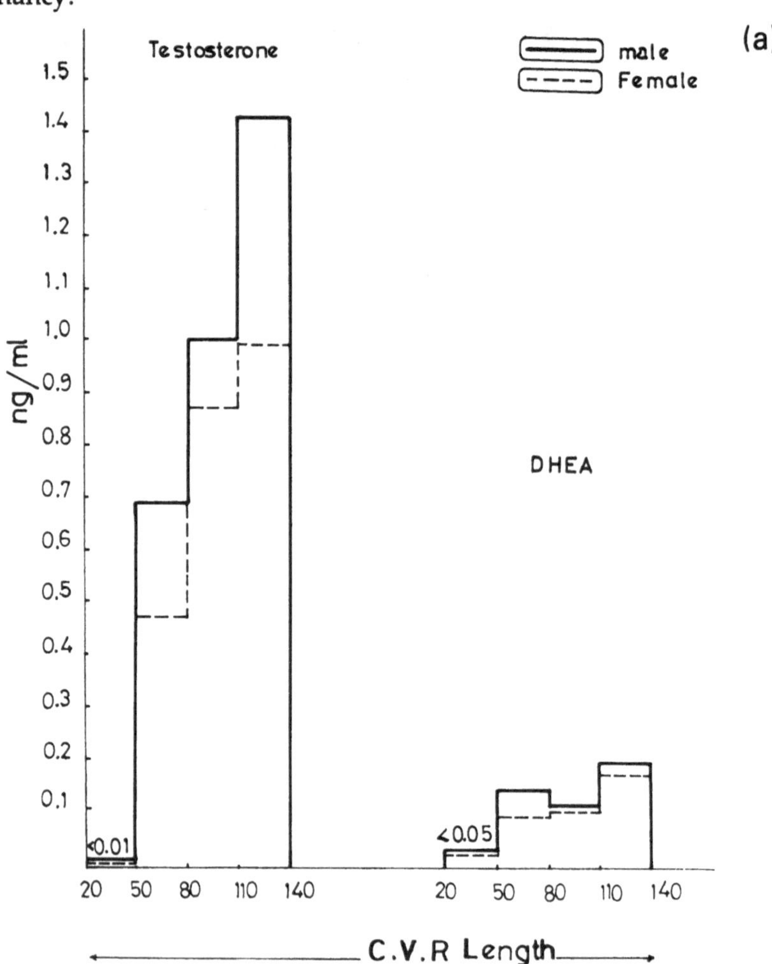

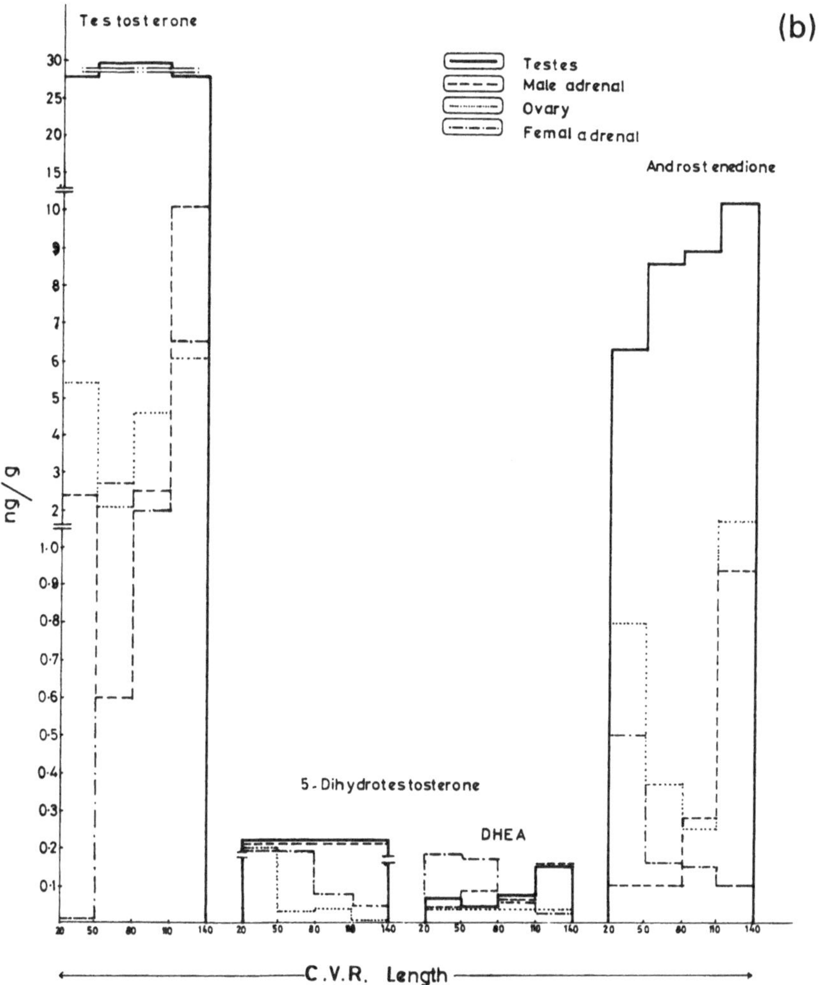

Figure 1 (*a*) Testosterone and dihydroepiandrosterone (DHEA) levels in fetal plasma. (*b*) Androgen levels in fetal testes, ovary and adrenal gland

DISCUSSION

There is no available literature on fetal camel hormone. For this reason, it was thought that comparison of the results with that of other animal fetuses would be rather interesting.

Our data on androgens agree with the data from studies designed to test the capacity of the fetal testes to produce androgens and to respond to gonadotrophin stimulation. Male phenotype sexual differentiation in mammals depends upon testosterone secretion by the fetal testes, and the testicular leydig cells of rhesus fetuses are steroidogenically active and can respond to gonadotrophin during gestation[2].

Our findings on an increase in testosterone, androstenedione and dehydroepiandrosterone levels reflect the findings that there is a high level of testosterone in lamb fetal plasma during late pregnancy until just prior to parturition[3]. Testosterone in cord blood from pregnant monkey in high concentrations was found in the presence of the male fetus (these high levels were abolished by castration) in both sexes, and there was an increase in the plasma testosterone between day 141 and 163 of pregnancy[4]. The rhesus fetus has a well-developed fetal adrenal cortex which is presumably the source of androstenedione and dehydroepiandrosterone sulphate present in fetal plasma in relatively high concentration[5].

It is apparent that in camel, the various components of the reproductive endocrine system are structurally complete quite early in fetal life. Furthermore, it could be hypothetically assumed that androgens were secreted from testes, adrenal glands of the male fetuses; and from the ovary and adrenal glands of the female fetuses.

References

1. Abraham, G.E. (1977). *Handbook of Radioimmunoassay*. Vol. 5. pp. 591–656. (California: Radioassay System Laboratories)
2. John, A.R. and Walliam, E.E. (1981). Testicular hormone production in foetal rhesus macaques. In Miles, J.N. and John, A.R. (eds.) *Fetal Endocrinology*. pp. 255–67. (New York: Academic Press)
3. Strott, C.A., Sundel, H. and Stahlman, M.T. (1977). Maternal and fetal plasma progesterone, cortisol, testosterone and 17β-estradiol in preparturient sheep. Response to fetal ACTH infusion. *Endocrinology*, **95**, 1327
4. Resko, J.A., Malley, A., Bogley, D. and Hess, D.L. (1973). Radioimmunoassay of testosterone during fetal development of the rhesus monkey. *Endocrinology*, **93**, 156
5. Liggins, G.C. (1981). Endocrinology of parturition. In Miles, J.N. and John, A.R. (eds.) *Fetal Endocrinology*. pp. 211–37. (New York: Academic Press)

43
The concentrations of corticosteroids in the plasma and tissues of the one-humped camel fetus

S.A.F. EL-MOUGY, F.B.S. WEHAISH and Y.M. RADWAN

INTRODUCTION

Although inadequate information exists on the reproductive events in the camel, there is none available on camel fetal endocrinology. A major link in the study implicating the ovine fetus in the initiation of parturition is the change in cortisol concentration in fetal plasma seen during late pregnancy. Evidence that spontaneous parturition in sheep includes an increase in the activity of the fetal pituitary–adrenal axis exists in the finding that the adrenal gland of the fetal lamb grows markedly in the last 10 days[1].

Fetal endocrine activity in early pregnancy is primarily related to the differentiation of the gonads and the psychosexual development of the brain. In late pregnancy, fetal endocrine activity initiates parturition and stimulates a variety of maturational changes that improve the chances of newborn survival[2].

Thus the present report measures the contribution of the adrenal gland of the one-humped camel fetus during prenatal development in the production of corticosteroids.

MATERIALS AND METHODS

Samples of blood and adrenal cortex tissue were obtained from fetuses.

(a)

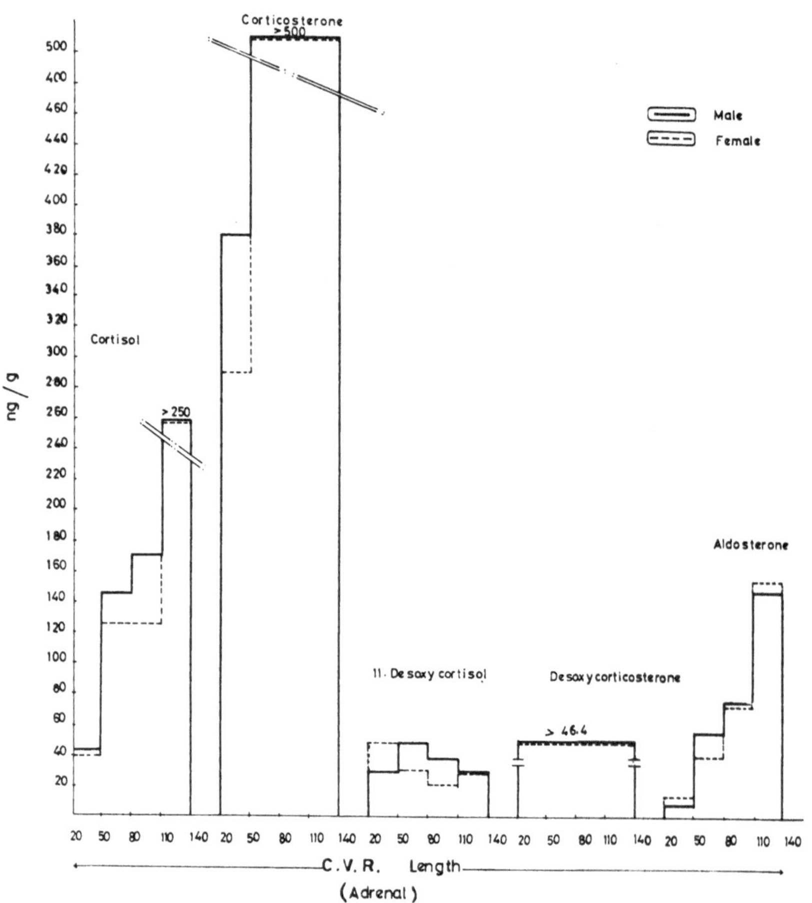

The samples were grouped according to the cranio-vertebral–rump (CVR) length of the fetus[3]. Blood samples were collected in heparinized plastic tubes and immediately centrifuged at 4°C at 4000 rpm for 30 minutes, then stored at −20°C until the day of assay. The adrenal cortex was kept at −20°C until used for hormonal assay. Cortisol, corticosterone, 11-desoxycortisol, desoxycorticosterone and aldosterone were estimated in plasma and adrenal cortex by RIA[4].

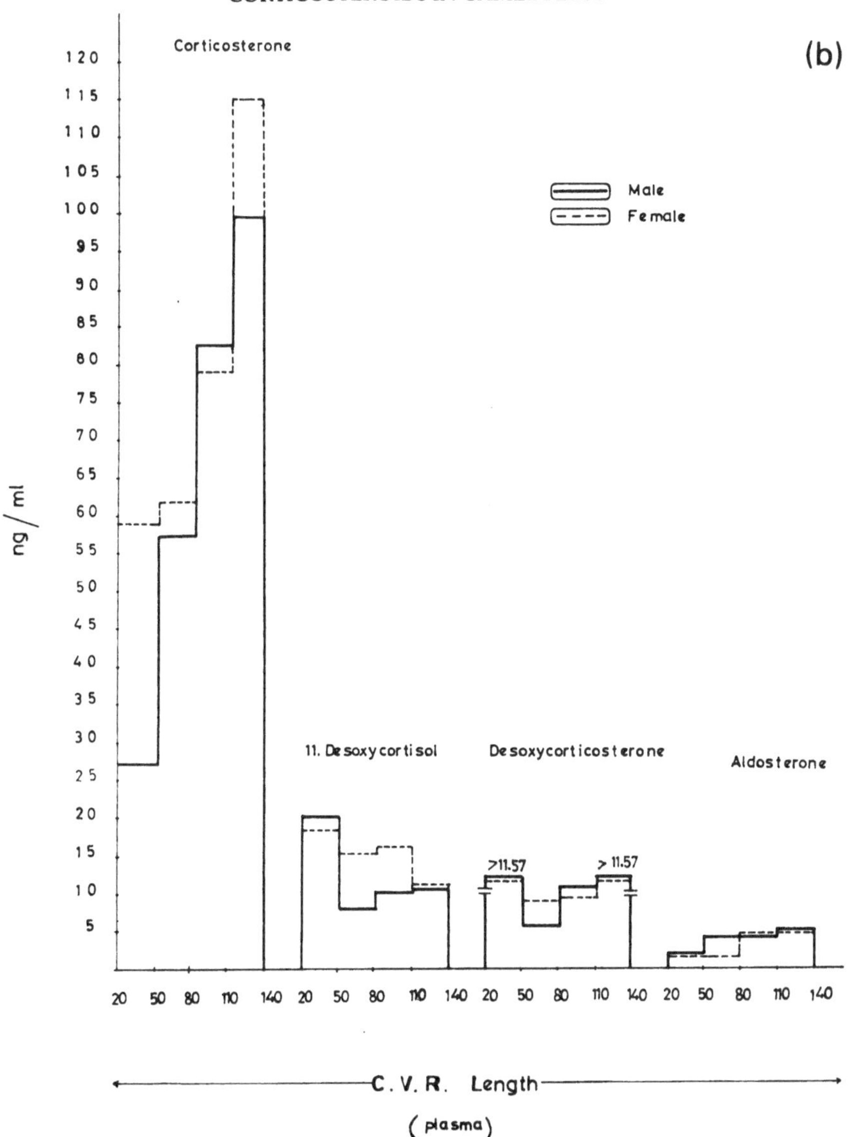

Figure 1 Concentration of corticosteroids in adrenal cortex (*a*) and plasma (*b*) of camel fetuses

RESULTS

Concentration of corticosteroids in the plasma and adrenal cortex are shown in Figure 1. Generally, a gradual significant increase in the level of corticosteroids with the development of the fetuses were observed, except for a slight decrease in the level of 11-desoxycortisol.

DISCUSSION

Corticosteroid concentrations of the one-humped camel fetus have not been described, so a comparison of the present findings must be made with other animal species.

The present work showed a gradual increase of corticosteroid levels in the plasma and adrenal glands with the development of the one-humped camel fetus. This result reflects the findings in other species[5,6]. The hypothesis that there is a marked stimulation of the fetal adrenal cortex, through factors such as ACTH stimulation of steroid secretion in human and monkey fetal adrenal tissue, prolactin, human chorionic gonadotrophin, and melanocyte stimulating hormone[7], remains to be confirmed in fetal camel endocrinology. The fetal adrenals have been found to be capable of carrying out the complete set of reactions in the conversion of acetate to cortisol and aldosterone by week 20 of human gestation. *In vivo,* the decrease in cortisol production would lead to an increase in ACTH secretion and the adrenal cortical growth would be stimulated[8]. However, despite the recognition that the hypothalamic–pituitary axis must be involved, there is controversy over the factors responsible for the accelerated secretion of fetal adrenal hormone with advancing gestation; another important question is the source of the substrate utilized by the fetal adrenals for steroid hormone biosynthesis.

References

1. Comline, R.S. and Sliver, M. (1961). The release of adrenaline and noradrenaline from
   the adrenal gland of the foetal sheep. *J. Physiol.*, **156**, 424–44
2. Miles, J.N. and John, A.R. (1981). *Fetal Endocrinology, ORRC. Symposia on Primate Reproductive Biology*. p. 3. (New York: Academic Press)
3. Safa, O.A.F. (1962). *Prenatal Development of some Endocrine Glands. The Thyroid Gland of*
   Camel Embryos. MSc Thesis, Faculty of Agriculture, Ein Shams University, Egypt
4. Abraham, G.E. (1977). *Handbook of Radioimmunoassay*. Vol. 5. pp. 591–656. (California:
   Radioassay System Laboratories)
5. Patrick, J.E., Cjallis, J.R.G., Johson, P., Rabunson, J.S. and Thorburn, G.O. (1976). Cortisol in amniotic fluid of rhesus monkey. *J. Endocrinol.*, **68**, 161–62
6. Jaffe, R.B., Seron-Ferre, M., Crickard, K., Koritnik, D., Mitchell B.F. and Huhtamiemi, I.I. (1981). *Rec. Prog. Horm. Res.*, **37**, 41
7. Miles, J.N. and Scott, W.W. (1981). Regulation of fetoplacental steroidogenisis in rhesus macaques. In Miles, J.N. and John, A.R. (eds.) *Fetal Endocrinology*. pp. 65–94. (New York: Academic Press)
8. John, W.R. (1981). Development and function of the human fetal adrenal cortex. In Miles, J.N. and John, A.R. (eds.) *Fetal Endocrinology*. (New York: Academic Press)

44 Treatment with progesterone in threatened abortion and low level of serum progesterone. A double-blind randomized trial

F. SØNDERGAARD, B.S. OTTESEN, G.U. DETLEFSEN, S.C. PEDERSEN, L. SCHIERUP and P.E. LEBECH

The production of progesterone by the corpus luteum is indispensable in the maintenance of early pregnancy[1]. Lute ectomy before the 6th–7th week of gestation leads to abortion, while replacement therapy with progesterone prevents abortion[1]. It has therefore been suggested to treat threatened abortion with progesterone. Synthetic gestagens are of no use for this purpose because of the luteolytic and teratogenic effects[2–4]. The aim of the present study has therefore been to evaluate the effect of genuine progesterone suppositories (200 mg three times daily) on early threatened abortion with serum progesterone values less than 33 nmol l^{-1}.

One hundred and forty-three patients with threatened abortion during the first 10 weeks of pregnancy entered this double-blind clinical controlled study after written informed consent and after the study was approved by the local Ethical Committee for Copenhagen, Denmark. Forty-two patients had serum progesterone values less than 33 nmol l^{-1}. Twenty-three patients were treated with progesterone and 19 received placebo. Blood samples were collected for the measurement of progesterone (Figure 1), human placental lactogen, oestradiol and hCG. Replacement therapy with genuine progesterone was without effect on the number of abortions compared with the placebo group (Table 1). The treatment with progesterone induced a significant increase in the serum progesterone values.

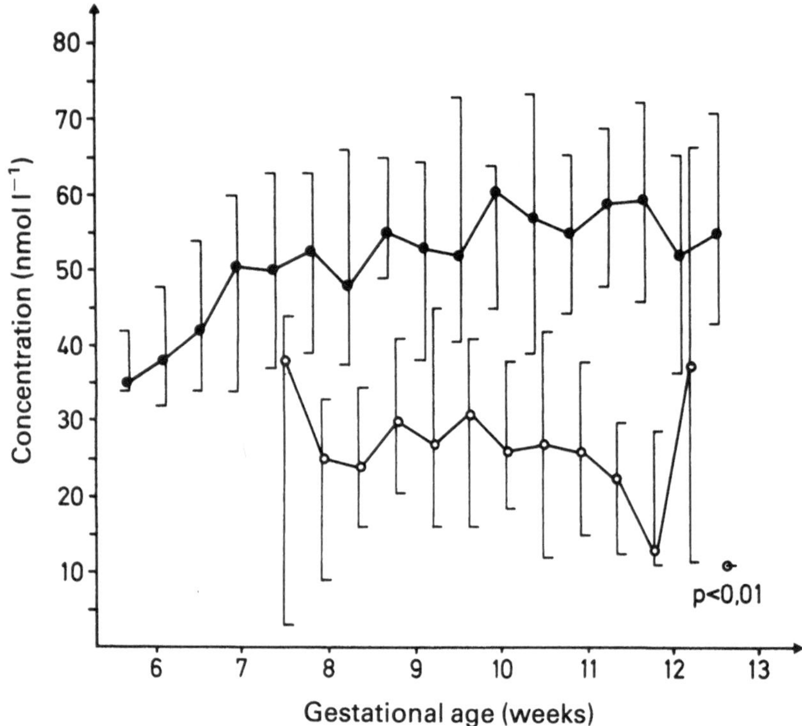

Figure 1 The relationship between serum progesterone and gestational age in threatened abortion (n = 143). In the patients receiving progesterone suppositories the blood samples were collected immediately before the administration of a suppository. Progesterone was measured by a competitive protein binding assay.
•—• = Patients receiving progesterone and not undergoing abortion;
o—o = patients receiving progesterone and undergoing abortion

The present observation does not lend support to the hypothesis that progesterone-replacement therapy is rational in the treatment of threatened early abortion with low serum progesterone.

Table 1 The number of abortions in 42 women with threatened abortion and a serum progesterone value less than 33 nmol l^{-1}, treated with genuine progesterone or placebo in a double-blind, prospective, clinical controlled trial

Group	*Non-abortions*	*Abortions*	*Total*
Placebo	2	17	19
Treatment	6	17	23
Grand total	8	34	42

Statistical calculations: Fischer's exact test, not significant (p>0.2).

References

1. Csapo, A.I. and Pulkkinen, M. (1978). Indispensability of the human corpus luteum in the maintenance of early pregnancy luteectomy evidence. *Obstet. Gynecol. Survey*, **33**, 69
2. Johansen, E.D.B. (1971). Depression of progesterone levels in plasma in women treated with synthetic gestagens after ovulation. *Acta Endocrinol.*, **68**, 779
3. Cortés-Gallegos, V. (1973). Agentes luteoliticos y reproduction. *Gac. Med. Méx.*, **106**, 259
4. Heinonen, O.P., *et al.* (1977). Cardiovascular birth defects and antenatal exposure to female sex hormones. *N. Engl. J. Med.*, **296**, 67

Index